Multidisciplinary Experiences in Renal Replacement Therapy

Edited by Ane C.F. Nunes

Published in London, United Kingdom

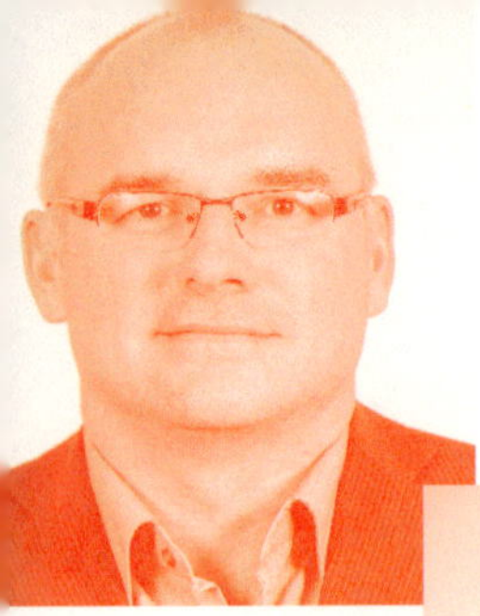
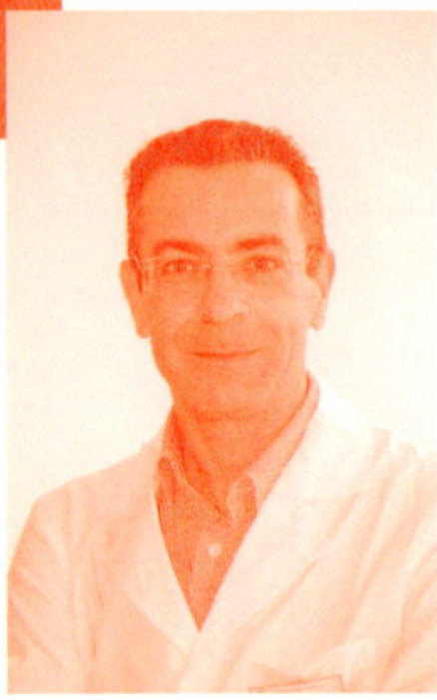
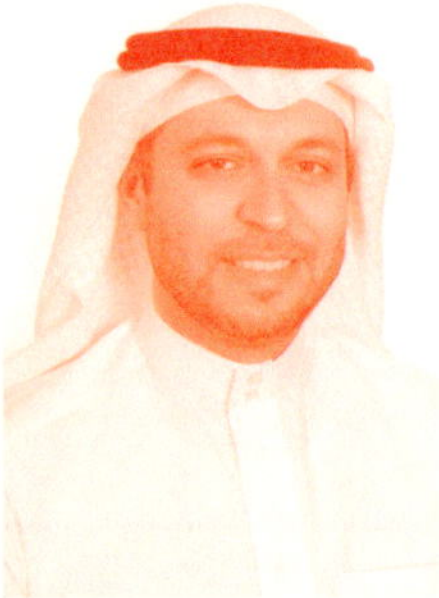
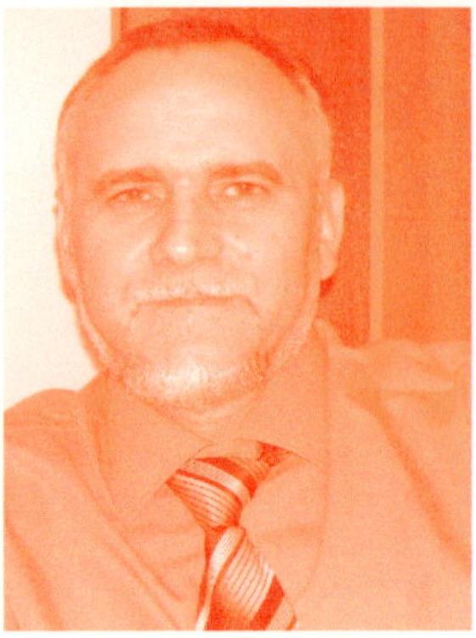
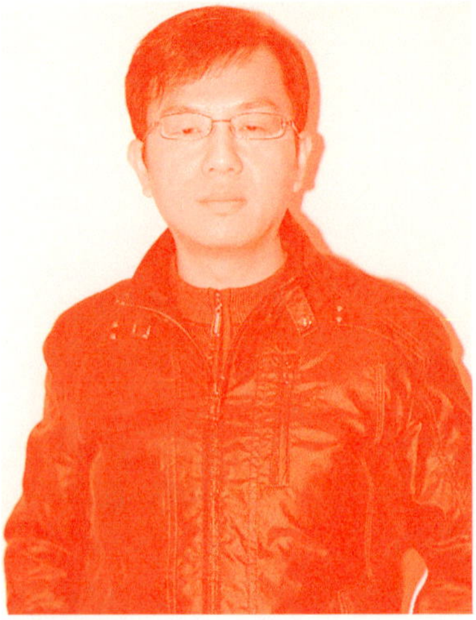
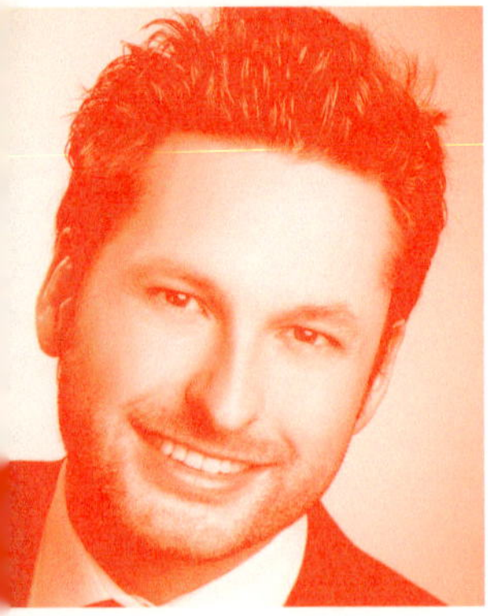
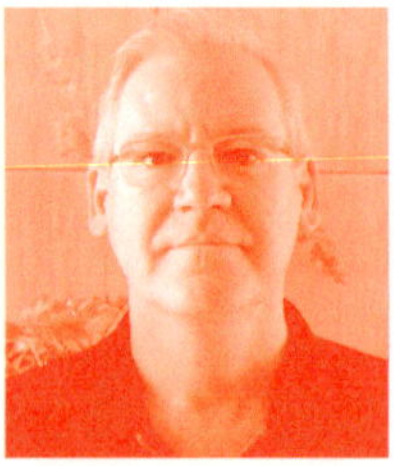

IntechOpen

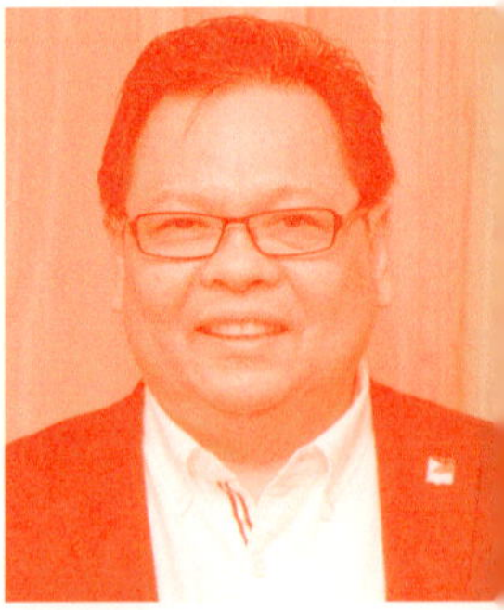
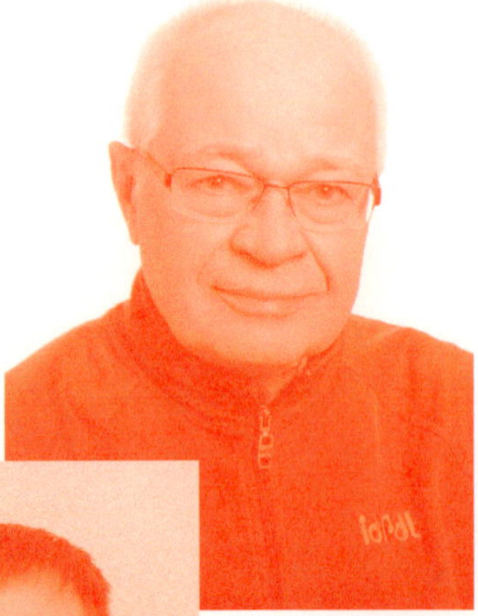
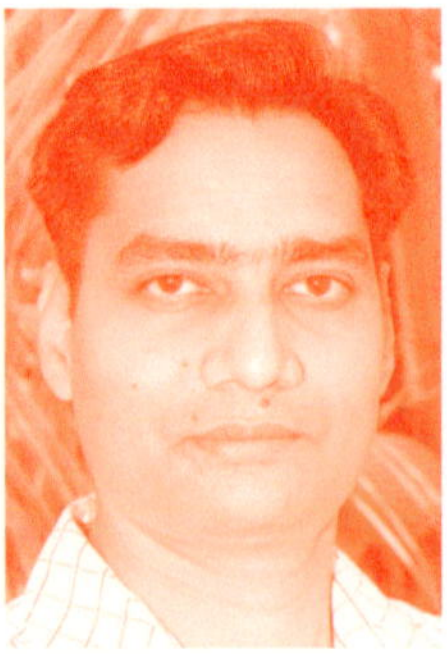
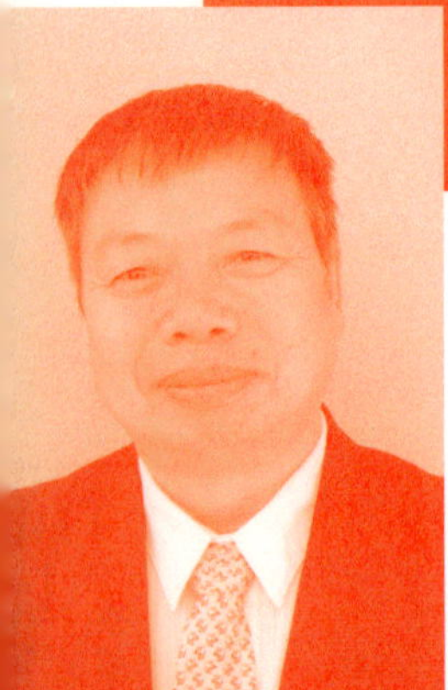
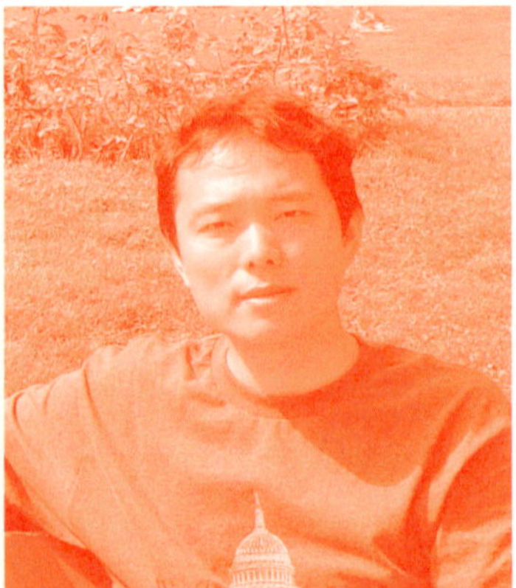
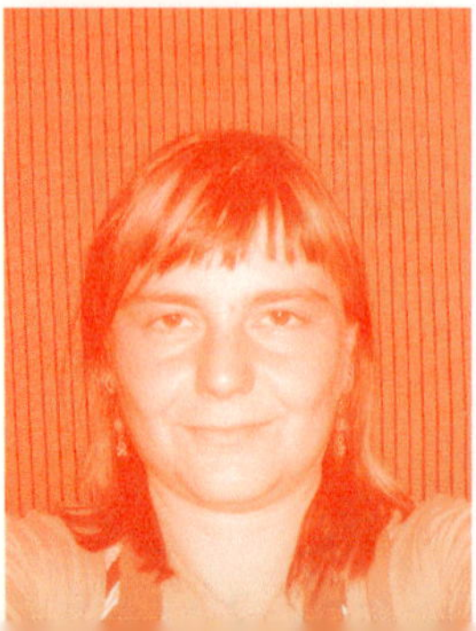

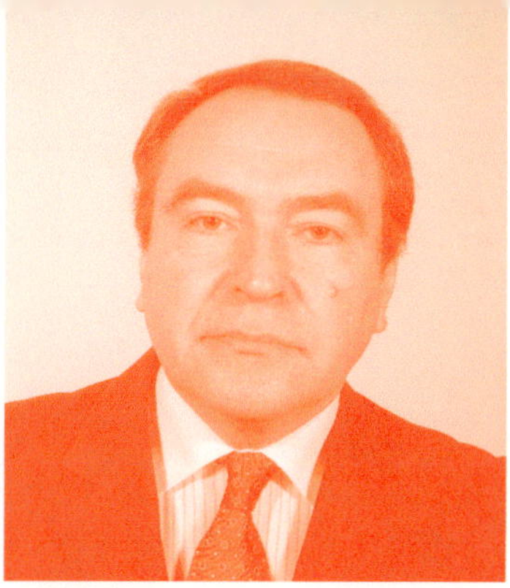
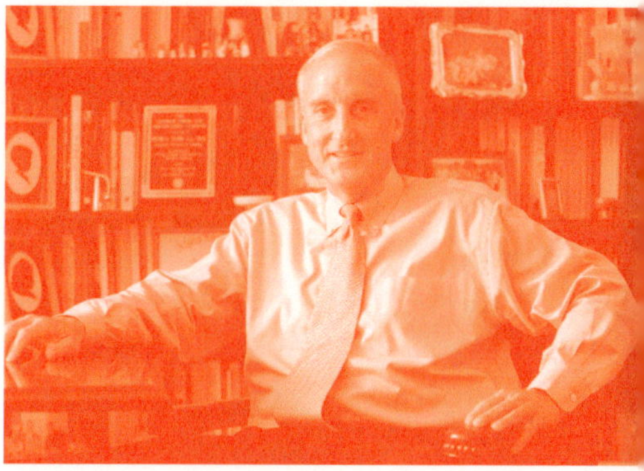
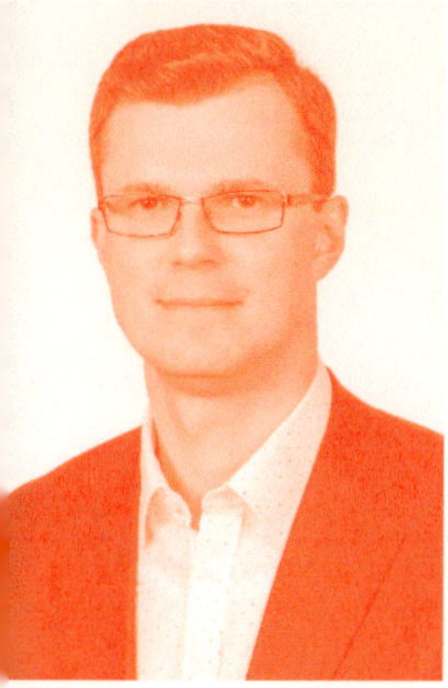
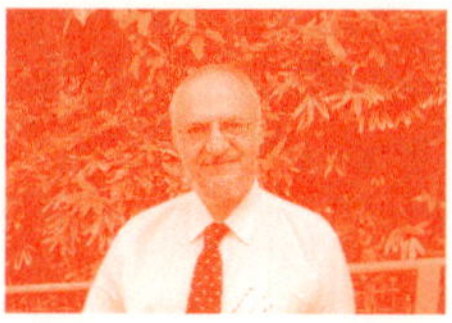
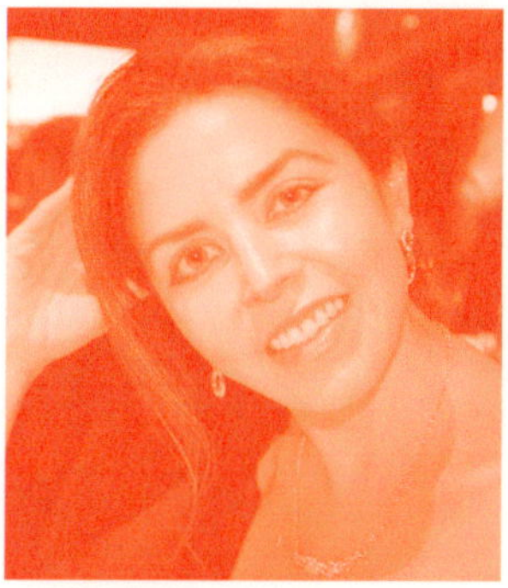

Supporting open minds since 2005

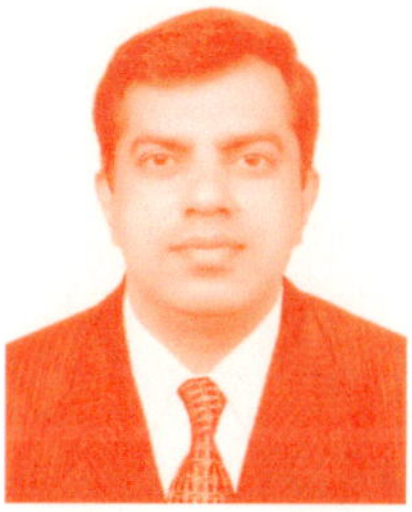
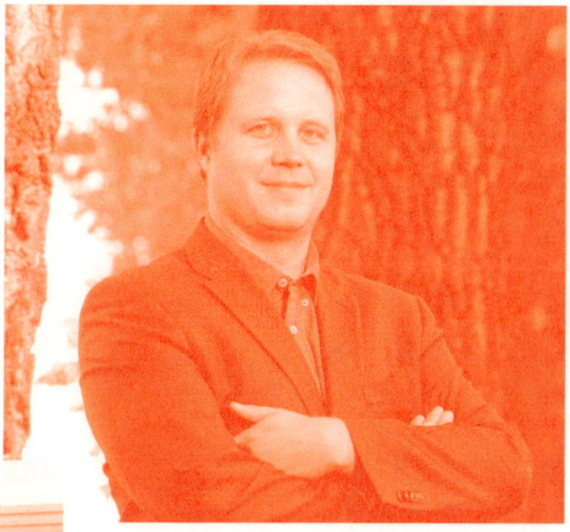
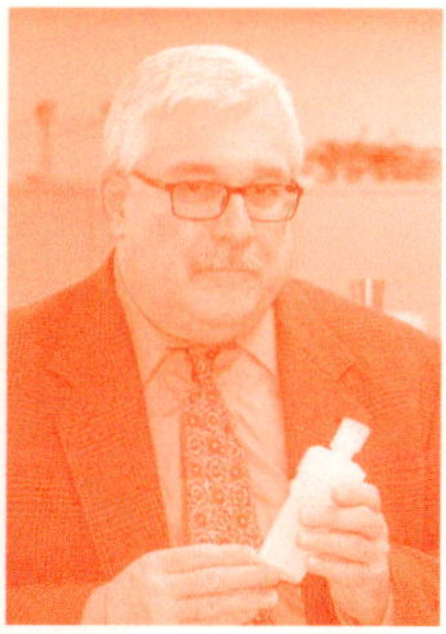
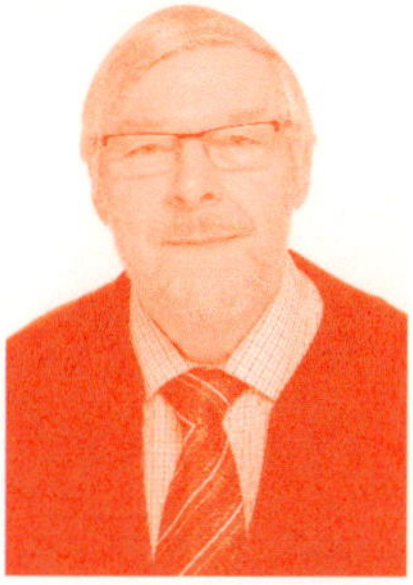
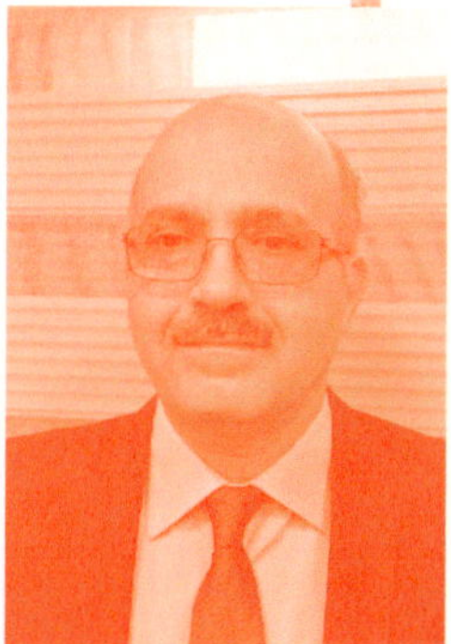
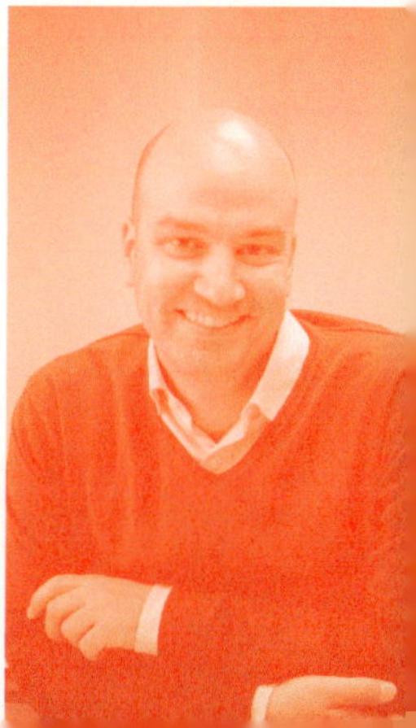
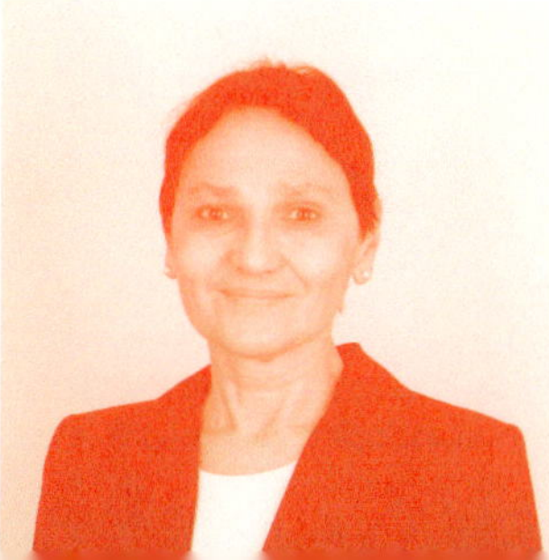

Multidisciplinary Experiences in Renal Replacement Therapy
http://dx.doi.org/10.5772/intechopen.90960
Edited by Ane C.F. Nunes

Contributors
Dhanya Michael, Joseph S. Fidelis, Sijo Joseph Pakalomattom, Renata De Paula Faria Rocha, Rayane Alves Moreira, Ana Luiza Gonçalves Moura, Moema da Silva Borges, Evgeny Shutov, Natalia Filatova, Xiangling Wang, Hanny Sawaf, Angelika L. Erwin, Fang Zhao, Tushar J. Vachharajani, Vaidehi A. Patel, Alexey E. Khrulev, Irina V. Belova, Irina V. Soloveva, Anna G. Tochilina, Natalya A. Shiyanova, Anastasiya A. Nikitina, Natalya S. Khruleva, Raid D. Hashim, Arturo Rafael Vizcarra

First published in London, United Kingdom, 2022 by IntechOpen
IntechOpen is the global imprint of INTECHOPEN LIMITED, registered in England and Wales, registration number: 11086078, 5 Princes Gate Court, London, SW7 2QJ, United Kingdom
Printed in Croatia

British Library Cataloguing-in-Publication Data
A catalogue record for this book is available from the British Library

Additional hard and PDF copies can be obtained from orders@intechopen.com

Multidisciplinary Experiences in Renal Replacement Therapy
Edited by Ane C.F. Nunes
p. cm.
Print ISBN 978-1-83962-662-3
Online ISBN 978-1-83962-663-0
eBook (PDF) ISBN 978-1-83962-664-7

For EU product safety concerns:
IN TECH d.o.o., Prolaz Marije Krucifikse Kozulić 3, 51000 Rijeka, Croatia, info@intechopen.com or visit our website at intechopen.com.

Meet the editor

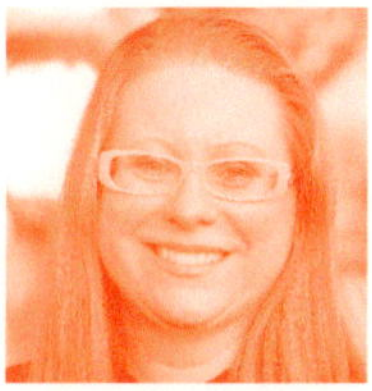

Dr. Ane C.F. Nunes is a geneticist with a master's degree and Ph.D. in Medical Sciences and Nephrology from the Federal University of Rio Grande do Sul (UFRGS), Brazil. She has post-doctoral experience in renal physiology from the Federal University of Rio de Janeiro (UFRJ), Brazil; clinical medicine and nephrology from the University of São Paulo (USP), Brazil; and nephrology and hypertension from the University of California, Irvine (UCI), USA. She is a Professor of Medical Genetics, Human Genetics, and Molecular Biology. Her research interests include human genetic diseases and cellular and molecular biology applied to nephrology, biochemistry, and microbiology with projects in the following subjects: inflammatory markers, molecular diagnosis, DNA polymorphisms, chronic kidney disease (CKD), polycystic kidney disease (PKD), Fabry disease, rare diseases, cellular and murine models for CKD, RNA processing, fluorescent image analysis, nanoparticles development, and nanomedicine.

Contents

Preface

Renal failure is a many-sided clinical state that normally progresses to kidney chronic disease (CKD). Renal replacement therapy (RRT) is a set of techniques applied to replace the capacity of blood filtration, which is completely lost in end-stage renal disease (ESRD).

This book brings a multidisciplinary approach to RRT in its three sections, from qualitative analysis to technical and clinical reviews.

Section I, "Health and Wellness," includes two chapters that summarize crucial aspects of promoting the health and wellness of ESRD patients. In Chapter 1, Michael et al. present important aspects of Quality of Life (QoL) and exercise for patients. This chapter refers to the definitions and perceptions used as markers for QoL as a tool to be added to the nursing routine. Chapter 2, by Moreira et al., discusses "hope" as a multidimensional concept and its application in the follow-up of patients undergoing hemodialysis and peritoneal dialysis.

Section II, "Hemodialysis Routine and Patients Care," includes three chapters. Chapter 3, by Patel, discusses vascular access, from the role of radiology in technical practice to the potential early and late complications related to this procedure. Chapter 4 by Vizcarra reviews vascular accesses for hemodialysis. Chapter 5 by Rocha examines patient safety in hemodialysis and discusses some key aspects for reducing the risk of unnecessary harm related to hemodialysis.

Section III, "Renal-Associated Diseases and Clinical Biomarkers," includes four chapters. Chapter 6 by Khrulev et al. reviews cerebrovascular disorders in both pre-dialysis and RRT patients from a pathophysiologic point of view and discusses clinical endpoints among patients at two-year follow-up. Chapter 7 is a remarkable assessment of Fabry disease (FD) by Wang et al. This X-linked lysosomal storage disorder has an important impact on renal function. Some FD patients are submitted to enzymatic replacement therapy while undergoing RRT and the understanding of this genetic disease is crucial for better clinical management. In Chapter 8, Hashim reviews the prognostic value of serum parathyroid hormone (PTH) in patients with ESRD, focusing on plasma PTH level parameters in CKD. Finally, Chapter 9 by Shutov and Filatova summarizes cardiorenal syndrome in patients on RRT.

Clinical routines are increasingly focused on the translational scenario of health sciences. Practically all procedures of a medical clinic depend on the participation of professionals from different areas of health. Therefore, *Multidisciplinary Experiences in Renal Replacement Therapy* brings together studies from different perspectives on RRT.

As an editor, I am honored to have organized the studies included in this book. I thank all the contributing authors and the staff at IntechOpen for their commitment and dedication to the project.

Ane C.F. Nunes, Ph.D.
University of California,
Irvine, USA

Section 1

Health and Wellness

Chapter 1

Effect of Exercise on Health-Related Quality of Life in Patients with End-Stage Renal Disease

Dhanya Michael, Joseph S. Fidelis and Sijo Joseph Pakalomattom

Abstract

Chronic kidney disease (CKD) is becoming more common around the world. Chronic kidney disease (CKD) is linked to a wide range of other health problems, such as diabetes, hypertension, stroke, and pulmonary illness. Patients with CKD tend to lead sedentary lives for a variety of reasons. Dialysis patients, on the other hand, are much less active than the general population. All of these factors raise the likelihood of future morbidity and mortality, while also lowering the overall quality of life for people who are ill (HRQoL). Regular physical activity (PE) has been shown to increase overall well-being and HRQoL. Here, we discuss several PEs and their effects on CKD patients' physical fitness, function, and HRQoL, as well as the significance of haematocrit normalisation and the influence on their serum phosphorus levels. We have discussed the advantages of PE for this particular population of individuals as well as the side effects of intradialytic PE. There have also been discussions on factors that contribute to impaired physical function in CKD patients and the impact of PEs on different bodily systems.

Keywords: chronic kidney disease, end-stage renal disease, health-related quality of life, physical exercise, quality of life

1. Introduction

Health and QoL (quality of life) have different meanings to different people. Despite the fact that health has an impact on life happiness, health is simply a minor factor. As a result, health is seen as a component of QoL [1]. Perceived QoL refers to how people view and evaluate their quality of life. Subjective quantification refers to measuring how satisfied and happy you are with many aspects of your life, such as your health [2]. It is a notion that advocates quantifying your own life experience subjectively.

Health-related QoL (HRQoL) is a subgroup of QoL that is most affected by health or treatment [1]. Furthermore, either disease-specific or generic tools estimate it. It collects data on patients' knowledge about specific areas of health, such as HIV-QL31 or EORTC QLQ-C30, that are affected by a specific disease, whereas the latter measures general well-being that is applicable to all health states, including healthy individuals such as the 36-Item Short-Form (SF-36®) Survey or the EuroQoL 5 Domain (EQ-5D) tool.

IntechOpen

Chronic diseases have become more common during the previous few decades. This is because the population is getting older, medical technology is improving, and infectious diseases are being better prevented and managed. Consequently, a higher proportion of people suffer from long-term disorders that impair their HRQoL. Chronically ill adults, such as those with hypertension, diabetes, coronary heart disease, congestive heart failure, chronic obstructive pulmonary disease, and arthritis, have lower HRQoL than healthy adults. Co-existing diseases reduce HRQoL even further [3].

Chronic diseases affect a range of HRQoL indicators, such as pain, general health, mental health, social function, and sleep, and a lower HRQoL may be the result. The primary care services supplied may have an impact on these other industries (e.g. mental health counselling, pain medication, and self-management education to aid in performing routine functions). HRQoL estimates, including complicated processes such as intervention dose–response relationships, might therefore play an important role in evaluating primary care services. An assessment of HRQoL in individuals with chronic conditions may also help raise awareness of the significance of providing high-quality care to all patients. HRQoL considerations are an important part of providing patient-centred comprehensive care, and this approach can help patients by improving their self-management skills. HRQoL. HRQoL estimates can be used for a variety of purposes, including patient-physician contact, programme design, and support services. A simple HRQoL assessment can make a big difference in a patient's quality of life [3].

Chronic kidney disease is defined as renal failure that lasts more than 90 days (CKD). It is quite common, affecting between 2.5 and 11.2% of adults in Asia, Australia, Europe, and the United States. If untreated, albuminuria can proceed to end-stage renal disease (eGFR 15 mL/min/1.73 m^2 and urine albumin >300 mg/g), necessitating a kidney transplant or the usage of MHD/PD (RT). The annual healthcare cost for persons with end-stage renal disease (ESRD) exceeds $1 trillion, indicating a considerable financial burden [4]. In India, HD is expected to cost INR 29,852 per month while peritoneal dialysis will cost INR 28,763 per month [5]. According to another study, sustaining individuals with ESRD costs INR 2,13,144 per year [6].

HRQoL deteriorates as CKD progresses in patients with ESRD, and is usually harmed as a result of lifestyle and dietary constraints, disease-related complications, multiple comorbidities, polypharmacy, dialysis-related side effects, rapid ageing, and a uraemic milieu [7]. Poor HRQoL has been associated with an increased risk of hospitalisation and mortality [7, 8], and therefore, attempts to enhance it are necessary for more than just obtaining a good HRQoL target.

Patients with CKD who do not require dialysis or HD are urged to participate in physical activity (PE), which should include 30 minutes of aerobic exercise (AE) on most days of the week [9, 10]. Despite these recommendations, physical activity levels, activity-related energy expenditure, and daily step count in CKD patients on MHD were all shown to be comparable to those of a sedentary lifestyle. In people with CKD and RT, a growing body of evidence demonstrates that regular PE improves HRQoL, the cardiovascular (CV) system, aerobic fitness, and walking capacity.

Physical activity benefits patients with CKD, especially those with end-stage renal illness, according to these data (ESRD).

2. Definitions

Quality of life (QoL): This is a phrase used to describe how well a person feels about their position in life as it relates to the culture and value frameworks in which they live, as well as their personal goals, standards, expectations, and concerns.

Furthermore, QoL refers to an all-encompassing sense of well-being that includes both objective and individual-level weighted metrics of well-being in terms of emotions, physical health, social well-being, and material well-being [1].

HRQoL relates to how well a person functions and perceives their well-being in connection to their physical, psychological, and social health, and includes well-being traits that are linked to or influenced by the presence of sickness or treatment [1, 2].

Physical activity (PA) is any movement of the body that needs the expenditure of energy and is caused by the activation of skeletal muscles [11]. Because it encompasses all motor behaviour, including both routine and recreational activities, it is an essential lifestyle aspect for overall health and well-being [12].

Physical exercise (PE) is a subcategory of PA that includes motions that are pre-planned, structured, and repeated. One or more aspects of physical fitness are improved or maintained as a final or transitional goal [11]. Aerobic and anaerobic activities with a set frequency, duration, and intensity constitute one type of PE.

3. Types of physical exercises

Patients with CKD who have PE had better outcomes overall, as previously mentioned. These individuals were indicated for a wide range of PEs, including the ones listed below:

3.1 Aerobic exercise (AE)

Aerobic energy production efficiency improves and cardiorespiratory fitness improves after taking AEs. Walking, running, cycling, rowing, and swimming are all examples of low-impact exercise. There are numerous health benefits to doing this, including higher insulin sensitivity (IS), greater mitochondrial density, increased levels of antioxidant enzymes in the body, improved lung and immune system performance, and increased cardiac output [13]. Patients with chronic diseases benefit from AEs because they lower their blood pressure (BP) and increase their maximum oxygen intake. Aside from improving physical function and aerobic capacity, these treatments may also provide other benefits for the patients. CKD patients on haemodialysis who engage in regular aerobic physical activity see some improvement in their diminished functional capacity [14]. AE may improve renal function and quality of life in CKD patients [15]. In-between-session AEs have shown encouraging benefits [16–18].

3.2 Resistance exercise (RE)

All main muscle groups are used in RE, which uses weight or resistance to make the body's skeletal muscles contract. In addition to lowering glycated haemoglobin levels, it has been linked to improvements in CV, body mass, physical function, glycaemic control, insulin sensitivity, blood pressure, and lipid profiles. Comparatively, it has a lower risk of hypoglycaemia and blood glucose fluctuations [13]. In order to help patients achieve functional independence, the RE is designed to include activities and context-oriented practice in areas that are important to each patient. It targets the antigravity muscles in particular and aims for the greatest possible carryover into daily activities. Body weight, gravity, resistance bands, free weights, and a weight vest can all act as resistance [19].

3.3 Combined exercise (CE)

It incorporates elements of AE and RE in one module. With CE, health and general cardiovascular benefits can be optimised while minimising risk factors associated with sedentary lifestyles. Because of this, it leads to better blood pressure regulation as well as lower insulin and glucose levels, glycated haemoglobin, visceral adipose tissue, and microalbuminuria [13].

3.4 Flexibility and balance exercises

Individuals benefit from it because it stretches muscles and improves balance and postural stability, allowing them to move more freely during other workouts and in daily life. It is possible for these to be static (e.g. not bending the knees) or dynamic (e.g. high knees). Exercises that improve balance and save you from falling include balance training. If you want to walk backwards or heel-toe in a straight line, you can do so [13].

Patients with severe renal impairment benefit equally from resistance and balance exercises, which both increase physical activity and improve renal function. Thus, to enhance the therapy effects of exercise in dialysis patients, it is better to combine these components in a balanced fashion or to change them individually [20].

4. Physical exercise in chronic illness

4.1 General impact

An important risk factor for many chronic diseases is physical inactivity, which can be prevented and treated. Chronic physical inactivity has been linked to an increased incidence of adverse CV events and a greater death rate in patients with peripheral arterial disease and dialysis. Simple frequent physical activity can serve as a springboard for healthy living and deliver substantial health benefits [21].

Daily PA and PE, according to current studies, can help avoid chronic diseases (such as cardiovascular disease, type 2 diabetes, obesity, and cancer) and mortality, as well as serve as a primary disease prevention strategy. Patients with high blood pressure and known cardiovascular diseases can potentially benefit metabolically and cardiovascularly from moderate-intensity activities [22–24]. A reduction in mortality risk may also result from improved and sustained physical fitness over time [10]. When a chronic illness is diagnosed, including PA and PE in the disease management strategy, improves the patient's overall health. PA and regular PE improve QoL and lengthen life when used in disease prevention or treatment [25].

Pre-dialysis patients with severe CKD suffer from decreased physical function and performance due to a variety of factors, including renal function decline, arteriosclerosis, and chronic inflammation [26]. Pre-dialysis CKD patients with improved physical performance and higher PA levels have lower overall mortality and CVD risk [27]. Patients with CKD benefit greatly from exercise training, which includes both aerobic and resistance activities, as well as increased muscle strength and lower blood pressure (BP) [26]. PE also benefits dialysis patients' physical health by improving CV function, blood pressure, muscle strength, and nutritional status, as well as improving dialysis quality [28]. For HD patients, PA in everyday life has a greater impact on QoL than it does in the general population [29].

4.2 Effect on physiological parameters

Muscle mass, strength, IS, mitochondrial content, and regeneration capacity can all be improved with PA. It is common to employ resistance training to build muscle and improve overall strength. As a result, your muscles get bigger and stronger, while your overall fitness increases. This includes considerable gains in myofibre and whole-muscle growth, strength, quality, and physical performance, or the prevention of these decreases.

Patients with cardiovascular disease benefit from regular PE because it lowers blood pressure, reduces resting heart rate, and raises atherogenic marker levels while also enhancing physiological cardiac hypertrophy. There are many benefits to losing weight, including decreased visceral adiposity, lowered cholesterol, HDL-C, and blood pressure (BP), as well as improved maximum oxygen consumption (VO2max) through either diet or exercise alone, or a combination of the two. Workout has been found to improve glucose homeostasis, endothelial function, blood pressure (BP), and HDL-C levels regardless of weight without affecting weight. Those who are overweight or have type 2 diabetes are at greater risk of cardiovascular disease, and regular exercise reduces that risk or severity [30, 31].

Regular physical activity and/or aerobic fitness are linked to better IS performance. Insulin resistance may usually be ameliorated and, in some cases, completely reversed, using PE interventions. Both acute and chronic effects of PA on IS have been documented in the literature. Acute effects can be seen during and/or for up to 72 hours after a single bout of physical activity and are directly linked to it. If these bouts are repeated on a regular basis, long-term chronic IS enhancement occurs, resulting in better glucose management than what is generally seen in people who are less active. There appears to be a dosage response with an increase in PA of 500 kcal/week, reducing the incidence of T2DM by about 9% [32]. Exercise's ability to improve IS and glucose absorption in the elderly is important [33]. Having a healthy lifestyle that includes moderate-intensity aerobic activity and/or PA on 3–5 days a week for at least 30 minutes has been linked to better IS and glycaemic management.

PE enhances the peroxisome proliferator-activated receptor co-activator 1 in cardiomyocytes after both endurance and resistance exercise (PGC-1) [33]. By improving mitochondrial fatty acid oxidation (the primary substrate used by healthy myocardium), PE also improves ATP synthesisation performance. Preventing CV dysfunctions in obese people, through PE-induced improvements in mitochondrial function, Is well documented. The reconfiguration of the mitochondrial network (fusion, fission, and autophagy) that occurs during exercise has also been found to improve mitochondrial function/efficiency [33].

4.3 Effect on general well-being

Recent research reveals that physical activity (PE) provides a number of benefits for people of all ages, and that it improves psychological well-being and quality of life (QoL). Physical education (PE) boosts self-efficacy, task orientation, and perceived competence in youngsters. Physical activity has been related to improved health outcomes in both children and adults, including a more positive self-image and a better mood. Last but not the least, for the elderly, physical activity promotes security, social connections, and mental health [34].

PE increases one's quality of life by interacting with biological and psychological systems. Higher cerebral blood flow improves oxygen delivery to brain tissue and allows for more oxygen consumption. Other biological causes include decreased muscular tension and increased endocannabinoid receptor numbers in the bloodstream, among others. The changing amounts of neurotransmitters caused by the phenomenon of neuroplasticity may also have an impact on one's overall well-being. When someone has a traumatic brain injury, their levels of neurotransmitters such as serotonin and endorphins rise. By emphasising the sense of control, self-efficacy, and competency, PE boosts students' self-esteem and self-concept while also creating a positive social synergy [34].

The benefits of regular and moderate physical activity extend beyond improved general health to lowered coronary heart disease (CHD) risk. T2DM patients who have PE experience a drop in their blood sugar and systolic blood pressure, which reduces their risk of developing DM-related complications, dying from the disease, or suffering from a heart attack. Because it reduces weight, PE lowers the risk factors for developing type 2 diabetes. Physical inactivity is linked to obesity and diabetes mellitus (DM), as well as a higher incidence and mortality from cancer (e.g. breast, endometrial). So PA and PE are linked to improved well-being and lowered mortality risk [35].

4.4 Improving physical fitness and function

Exercise therapy improves fitness and reduces the risk of illness consequences in people with chronic diseases [36]. Regular PA has been shown in these cases to enhance the human physique, lipid profiles (e.g. by decreasing the levels of total cholesterol, raising HDL-C levels, and diminishing the low-density lipoprotein [LDL]-to-HDL ratios), glucose homeostasis, autonomic tone, IS, coronary blood flow and endothelial function; improve cardiac function; and reduce BP, systemic inflammation, and blood coagulation. Chronic inflammation is a prominent cause in the majority of chronic illnesses, according to high levels of inflammatory markers such as C-reactive protein, and PE has been found to help avoid them [37].

Premature death is reduced when one's physical fitness improves, whereas it is increased when one's fitness deteriorates. Even a little increase in physical fitness has been shown to lead to a considerable decrease in risk. The health status of previously inactive adults improved significantly when their physical fitness was modestly increased [37]. Regular physical exercise reduces weight gain, obesity, coronary artery disease, type 2 diabetes, and Alzheimer's disease over time [38].

Even in the absence of increases in aerobic fitness, an improvement in health status indices can be detected as PA levels rise. That is especially true in the elderly, where frequent PA can minimise the risk of chronic illness and impairment while having no discernible effect on conventional physiologic performance metrics such as oxidative potential and cardiac output. PA can improve musculoskeletal fitness as well as cardiovascular fitness. According to a growing body of evidence, improved musculoskeletal fitness is linked to greater overall health and a lower risk of chronic illness and disability.

Health-related quality of life and hospitalisation, surgical results, and death are all influenced by one's ability to execute fundamental physical duties. Patients on haemodialysis benefit from PA because it increases their bodily function and physical ability, which lowers their blood pressure and increases their oxygen intake to their maximum potential [39]. The number of 30-second sit-to-stand tests (STS) increased after exercise began, and the time it took to complete the 8-foot timed up-and-go tests decreased, with no evidence of exercise-related unpleasant sensations. Some patients underwent a low-intensity home walking programme, while others were assigned at random to a slower-moving control group [40]. As a result, PE helps people with CKD become more fit and functional.

4.5 Patients with CKD

According to a recent meta-analysis, exercise treatment improved eGFR while simultaneously lowering blood pressure, BMI, and systolic blood pressure in CKD patients who were not on dialysis. Short-term exercises have been shown to lower TG levels as well [41]. Another systematic review and meta-analysis on individuals with comparable conditions found that frequent exercise increased peak oxygen consumption more than standard treatment and improved physical and walking abilities [26].

The effectiveness of a systematic physical exercise programme in patients with HD was examined over the course of a long trial, which also looked at patient compliance and the study's clinical outcomes. Exercise ability, strength, and QoL improved significantly over the course of a year in individuals with high and moderate compliance [42]. Recent meta-analysis shows that exercise improves HRQoL and aerobic capacity in people with ESRD undergoing HD. Patients' physical conditions improved as a result of doing aerobic or combination exercises for eight to 52 weeks, three times each week, according to the authors [43].

5. Risks associated with physical inactivity in patients with CKD

5.1 Why to improve HRQoL in patients with ESRD?

Patients on dialysis, like those with cancer or heart failure, have lower HRQoL and quality of life than the general population [44]. Treatment for end-stage renal disease (ESRD) has advanced significantly, but mortality and morbidity remain high and the quality of life for those on dialysis is declining. A patient's well-being and survival chances are taken into account when a treatment plan's success is assessed. ESRD patients are more likely to die or be hospitalised if their quality of life (QoL) is low, according to new research [45].

Despite improvements in care outcomes such as dialysis adequacy (Kt/V), phosphorus management, and haemoglobin levels, HRQoL among dialysis patients has not changed much over the preceding 10 years. The quest for therapies to improve dialysis patients' HRQoL has been undertaken by a number of studies. Renal replacement therapy's primary goal is to improve HRQoL in dialysis patients by increasing patient satisfaction and by improving their overall prognosis [46].

Overall survival has been linked to a range of clinical outcomes, including HRQoL (health-related quality of life). HRQoL measures both mental and physical health. The prevalence of depression in dialysis patients (up to 30%) has been linked to hospitalisation and mortality [47, 48]. A better mental health status can be achieved with the appropriate management [49]. Identifying and assessing the mental health state of these people is so critical. Another reason for low HRQoL is a patient's worsening physical health. Patient's PA and physical function are typically impaired in dialysis patients. There is a link between reduced PA and physical performance on an on-going basis and symptoms of depression and anxiety, and dialysis patients with lower physical function have a lower chance of survival [50, 51]. Patients on haemodialysis who are in poor physical health 3 months after dialysis begins are more likely to die [52].

As a result of these findings, we feel that HRQoL in ESRD patients must be improved in order to boost functional ability, psychological status, and patient satisfaction, lower mortality and hospitalisation rates, and improve the overall prognosis of the patients.

5.2 Exercise in patients with ESRD

On the day of dialysis, dialysis patients are much less physically active than the general aged population, as they are sedentary throughout the process and suffer from post-dialysis weariness. On days when they are not receiving dialysis, dialysis patients are 17% less physically active than non-dialysis patients. With decreased physical activity comes several risks, such as catabolic disorders that can cause muscle loss and lead to sarcopenia, mitochondrial dysfunction, and other conditions such as anaemia, mineral disorders, protein energy loss, diabetes, neurological dysfunction, and cardiovascular dysfunction [20]. Dialysis patients may also be at risk for these conditions.

Better results are strongly linked to increased levels of physical activity and healthy exercise habits. In all DOPPS countries, independent of physical state or social circumstances, patients who regularly exercised more than once a week had superior outcomes, according to the Dialysis Outcomes and Practice Pattern Study (DOPPS) [53]. Patients on CKD and dialysis who receive PA had a decreased death rate [20]. In addition, dialysis patients who completed a median of around 4000 steps daily and had PA of more than 50 minutes per day had better outcomes [54]. A less sedentary lifestyle is related to the improved results even in CKD patients with various impairments [20].

5.3 Factors leading to poor physical function

Exercise is hindered by factors that prevent genuine clinical practice from following the evidence. A study conducted in the United Kingdom found some important characteristics linked to CKD patients' behavioural alterations. Their physical health (frailty, anaemia, and age-related problems) and mental health (fear of damage or worsening of their ailment) were hindering their ability to engage in regular physical activity. People with concurrent illnesses and CKD-related symptoms including weariness and joint discomfort rated this as the biggest challenge to doing enough exercise [55]. Fear of injury was one of the biggest psychological barriers to physical activity. Some patients' fears about exercise may stem from the fact that healthcare providers are not adequately informing them about the health benefits of physical activity [56]. Individuals wanted individualised guidance and support from their healthcare providers on safe and effective exercises for those with kidney disease.

Further research from Canada found that weariness, dyspnoea, and weakness were the most common barriers to PE in a patient-reported outcome study (PRO). Regardless of modality or age group, PE patients preferred to exercise at home (73%) using a combination of AE and RE (41%). Despite the fact that most research has shown good effects on biochemical indicators and the potential for reduced mortality, these PRO studies suggest that these hopeful results are less meaningful for dialysis patients and may not encourage them to adhere to an "exercise regimen." Instead, they are looking for ways to reduce exhaustion and regain energy so they can go about their regular activities normally. As a result, it is critical that we identify and address these challenges in order to ensure high levels of patient satisfaction. In other words, custom programmes must be approved in order to start and sustain regular PE adherence.

6. Exercise has an effect on patients with CKD

As stated previously, patients with CKD are less fit and functionally compromised. When compared to healthy persons, their aerobic capacity is about half as poor, and they have weak physical strength and mobility problems. They are more likely to suffer from many disorders. People often complain of back, hip, and leg discomfort, tiredness, and muscle weakness due to electrolyte imbalance and other reasons [57].

6.1 Muscle structure and function

After a six-month exercise programme in HD patients, histological testing revealed a 51% increase in type II fibres and a 29% increase in average fibre area. There was also an increase in capillary density and mitochondrial regeneration [58]. Cross-sectional fibre area increased by 46% after 6 months of AE treatment, although another study found a drop in the percentage of atrophic fibre types I, IIa, and x as a result (from 51, 58, and 62% to 15, 21, and 32%, respectively). The therapy also improved the capillary network in the muscles. After a 12-week intradialytic progressive RE, there was a rise in thigh muscle volume [59]. The increased mitochondrial number and greater rate of protein synthesis that come with strength PE may also result in an increase in aerobic capacity. PE A rise in calcium levels in the cell cytoplasm, a surge in ATP production, and the creation of reactive oxygen species are all associated with endurance training, according to research [60]. Changes in mitochondrial function can occur after a few weeks of physical exertion (PE), and the degree of change is inversely proportional to PE intensity.

When looking at the effects of PE on adult CKD patients, a systematic review found that it had a significant favourable impact on metrics such as walking capacity, CV dimensions, and physical fitness [14]. Studies on exercise's positive effects on cardiopulmonary function, muscle strength, and walking ability in people with CKD revealed a meta-analysis [61].

A recent systematic review and meta-analysis found that resistance training, rather than aerobic training, significantly increased leg mass. After undergoing RE, my grip and knee extension strength significantly increased. AE claims to have enhanced the STS short form, but there is not enough proof to back them up. The 6-minute walking test score and the median version of the STS test in the physical performance dimension were both improved by AE and RE [62]. High-intensity resistance (RE) training on dialysis patients may increase muscular growth and strength, especially in the trained muscles. If dialysis patients desire to improve their physical performance, they can use AE and RE.

6.2 Nutrition

There is an imbalance between the increased protein requirement and the inadequate dietary food intake caused by HD, which results in skeletal muscle loss in CKD patients. Increased protein synthesis and anabolism from regular PE may help to slow the rate at which people lose lean body mass as they age. On non-HD days, however, As found in aged adults, and HD patients have a lower muscle protein synthesis response to diet. Furthermore, combining physical exercise with a high-protein diet has been shown to help decrease or even stop muscle loss. When used in conjunction with RE, intradialytic nutritional supplements improve both body composition and muscle mass. With PE, nutritional supplementation has significantly stronger protein anabolic effects when taken orally. Increased phosphorylation of mRNA translational signalling proteins due to RE and whey protein intake leads to enhanced protein synthesis in untrained individuals. In addition, ingestion of whey protein after RE activates the mTOR signalling pathway in a dose-dependent manner [63]. Supplementing PE with proper energy sources such as carbohydrates, protein, vitamins and iron will help keep muscle protein breakdown under control. Due to the energy loss and decreased digestive function associated with dialysis, patients are advised to consume more protein (1.2 times) than the average person.

6.3 Cardiovascular function

Systematic PE protects heart tissue in ESRD patients and slows the progression of coronary artery disease by reducing myocardial oxygen demand and facilitating better perfusion. Inflammatory indicators are reduced, and endothelial function is improved as a result. The NO levels can be raised and coronary arteries and other vessels dilated in as little as a few weeks of PE practice. Chronic AE lowers heart rate, systolic and mean blood pressure, and both at rest and during submaximal activity, decreasing myocardial oxygen demand in those with CHD. Submaximal PE improves arterial compliance, lowers peripheral vascular resistance, and boosts cardiac output in HD patients. As a result of reduced sympathetic tone, these beneficial adaptations may be due to increased parasympathetic activity, decreased catecholamine levels, and decreased endogenous cardiac output stimulation. PE, particularly the AE, raises resting vagal tone while lowering sympathetic tone in both healthy people and those with kidney disease [63].

There are only a few studies showing that PE can help patients with left ventricular dysfunction by increasing myocardial contractility, ejection fraction, stroke volume, and left ventricular mass. Improvements in skeletal muscle performance are another evidence of PE's beneficial effect on heart function [64]. The ejection fraction increased significantly after 30 minutes of intradialytic AE at 60–70% of maximum heart rate, according to the results of study. It was discovered that pre- and post-training left ventricular ejection fractions were associated with VO2peak [64]. HD patients who participated in an outpatient exercise training programme saw similar improvements in heart function [65]. Finally, long-term exercise helps hypertensive HD patients regulate their blood pressure and lowers their mortality rate [43, 66].

6.4 Glycaemic control and insulin resistance

With AE, you will have better IS and less IR. RE also lowered blood glucose levels, indicating that it could be a viable option for diabetic patients looking to improve their glycaemic control [13]. Muscle tissue insensitivity is the major source of IR, which is a common symptom of uraemia regardless of the kind of renal illness present. Regular physical activity enhances IS in healthy persons as well as those suffering from disorders linked to a sedentary lifestyle [67]. When establishing training programmes to enhance IR, total exercise length should be considered, with 3 hours of exercise per week being proven to be more effective than 2 hours [68]. Patients on HD may be more resistant to the effects of exercise on IR if they are in a uraemic setting. The results of a 12-month trial comprising 3 to 5 courses per week demonstrated that exercise has an impact on IR in this group.

A combination of CE and AE or RE is better at controlling blood sugar than either one alone. As a result of the CE increasing IS, adipose tissue loss, increased muscle mass, and decreased visceral and subcutaneous fat are all observed. When AE or RE is used alone, the glycated haemoglobin level improves. Patients who had CE, on the other hand, had better glycaemic control [13].

6.5 Renal function

Many studies have looked at how exercise affects CKD prognostic variables. Patients with CV illness and CKD demonstrated improved eGFR with exercise therapy, according to one study [69]. Another study [70] confirmed that patients with stage 3–4 CKD benefited from moderate-intensity exercise in terms of kidney function and BMI.

Meta-analysis of the impact of PE found that eGFR increased considerably in individuals with non-dialysis CKD, as did SBP, DBP, and BMI. PE had a rapid and considerable impact on TG levels (3 months). When it came to non-dialysis CKD patients, PE had no impact on SCr, TC, HDL-C, or LDL-C [41].

Kidney health benefits from exercise that includes both aerobic and resistance components. A meta-analysis of adult patients with CKD looked at renal function and discovered that combining exercise with medication significantly increased estimated glomerular filtration rate. The amount of creatinine in the blood was also reduced. These individuals' blood pressure has also reduced dramatically. There were no significant differences in proteinuria, cholesterol levels, physical composition, or quality of life between the groups.

6.6 HD efficiency

The inclusion of intradialytic AE significantly increased dialysis efficacy after the first month in a randomised controlled trial (RCT) and remained elevated throughout the programme [17]. Another RCT found that interdialytic mixed resistance and aerobic exercise enhanced physical performance in the sitting to standing, handgrip force task, time up and go, and 6-minute walk tests. Similarly, mini-nutritional assessment long-form scores increased considerably following the intervention period. The somatic and mental components of the QoL scale expanded significantly, but hospital anxiety and sadness decreased little. According to the results of the biological parameters, combined exercise reduced blood pressure while increasing HDL-C, LDL-C, and TGs levels throughout the body; however, there was no significant effect of intervention time on C-reactive protein, haemoglobin, albumin, or total cholesterol levels in the study participants' blood. In both the urea reduction ratio and the 6-minute walk test, aerobic and resistive training produced significant improvements. They dramatically increased dialysis efficiency and productivity [16].

6.7 Physical function and QoL

Regular exercise has been shown in a number of trials to help prevent CKD-related pulmonary function losses by strengthening respiratory muscles and increasing pulmonary function [71, 72]. After a year of training at home, participants with pre-dialysis CKD showed only minor gains in hand grip and knee extension strength [71]. Study after study found that older adults who were given more supervision gained more strength than older adults who were left alone, but these increases were often minimal [73]. Studies show that working out increases peak VO2 by 41% at the ventilatory threshold and 36% at the peak of activity. Ventilatory efficiency, on the other hand, was same between the two groups. The training groups did not differ in terms of strength or body composition; however, the 6MWT and 1STS showed improvement.

People with CKD had poorer HRQL even when they participate in exercise programmes despite evidence to the contrary [14]. Recent meta-analyses [43] reveal that physical activity improves aerobic capacity, walking ability, and HRQoL. The SF-36 domains of physical functioning, role physical, and role emotional all increased over time as a result of exercise training, resulting in remarkable improvements in overall health. After the exercise intervention, all five dimensions of Kidney Disease Quality of Life improved [74]. The EXITE (Exercise Introduction to Enhance Dialysis Performance) experiment found that MHD patients' functional status improved after a simple, personalised six-month home-walking programme. When compared to the normal treatment group, the exercise group exhibited a significant improvement in social interaction and cognitive performance, but the other 17 categories showed no significant differences [40]. There were five studies out of the 21 included in a meta-analysis that showed an increase in the SF-36 physical component score after exercise training, with a mean increase of 10%. In spite of the fact that the overall SF-36 physical component score changed little, the exercise group's physical component score increased by 43% [74].

7. Benefits of exercise

Regular PE in patients with CKD is associated with a myriad of health benefits, including physiological, psychological, and functional benefits.

7.1 Physiological benefits

Regular PE reduces CV mortality, hypertensive medication use, inflammatory markers (C-reactive protein); prevents muscle wasting; improves toxin removal by dialysis, exercise capacity, blood pressure control, lipid profile (increased HDL-C and reduced TG), haematocrit (prior to erythropoietin therapy), glycaemic control, serum albumin, nutritional summarise.

7.2 Psychological benefits

There is a link between regular physical activity and a better psychological profile (lower stress/anxiety/hostility/depression and increased engagement in pleasurable activities), perception of general and mental health, physical functioning, and vitality. Subjective weariness symptoms are reduced, as is the impression of physical pain, all at the same time [75–77].

7.3 Functional benefits

Regular physical exercise improves muscle strength, 6-minute walk distance, gait speed, sit-to-stand time, balance (which reduces the chance of falling), independence, and HRQoL [75–77].

8. Aerobic fitness and haematocrit (Hct) normalisation

Due to an increase in cardiac output and an improvement in muscles' innate ability to receive and use oxygen from the blood, physical activity has inherent benefits [78]. According to a meta-analysis, both moderate and intensive exercise trainings improve cardiorespiratory fitness and cardiometabolic health [79].

Patients with ESRD have a significant loss of fitness and functional competence [80], increasing their risk of death and limiting their ability to carry out everyday tasks [81, 82]. Renal anaemia is one of the most important variables that contribute to poor physical fitness [14]. Anaemia lowers oxygen carrying capacity, posing a barrier to maximum oxygen intake, PE capacity, and time to fatigue, particularly in those with ESRD [83].

Oxygen absorption can be viewed as an avenue for oxygen to get from the lungs to functioning tissues *via* systemic blood released by the heart during PE (physical exercise). Instead of being forced to deal with renal anaemia, recombinant erythropoietin was developed. A popular treatment for anaemia is erythropoiesis-stimulating agents (ESAs), which enhance QoL and cognitive function [84, 85], reduce left ventricular hypertrophy [86], and slightly increase maximum oxygen uptake in relation to haematocrit rise when used to treat anaemia [87]. Intradialytic PE, on the other hand, increases maximal oxygen absorption [88, 89] and has a cardioprotective effect [90]. PE, like ESAs, does not restore exercise ability in CKD patients to that of healthy people [24, 91]. Both of these treatments have been proven to improve maximum oxygen uptake and physical fitness, but they do not restore patients' fitness levels to those seen in the majority of sedentary people with normal renal function. Despite the fact that raising the haematocrit increases the blood's oxygen carrying capacity, other parts of the oxygen pathway remain intact, preventing the normalised haematocrit from providing any further health advantages. The ability of regular PE to give its maximal benefit is, on the other hand, restricted by the existence of anaemia. In a third situation, some components of dialysis or ESRD obstruct the regular oxygen pathway, which may be unaffected by either Hct normalisation or regular PE [92].

When compared to the numbers in the untrained anaemic phase, PE, Hct normalisation, or their combination leads in significantly increased maximal power and VO2. PE boosts cardiac output, peak tissue-diffusing capacity, and citrate synthase activity, but Hct normalisation boosts maximum arterial oxygen and arteriovenous oxygen difference. The maximal arteriovenous oxygen difference did not increase even when arterial oxygen levels increased in the combined phase, and they were the same as in healthy sedentary people [93]. As a result, it can be inferred that exercise and Hct normalisation have good effects but do not result in normalisation of exercise capacity in HD patients, which could be due to skeletal muscle anomalies.

9. Intradialytic exercise (IDE)

In order to urge patients to be more physically active, doctors often prescribe IDE (intermittent daily encouragement). It reduces fatigue, improves sleep quality, increases exercise tolerance, raises QoL, and even improves psychological status when used correctly. Furthermore, it has been proposed that IDE can boost dialysis's efficiency, which in turn reduces inflammation and boosts bone mineral density.

Because they may combine both aerobic and anaerobic elements into a single training session, the sit-to-stand test and the 6-minute walk test have been found to increase fitness. The depressive state index dropped significantly. The results of the QoL survey, with the exception of physiological discomfort, did not demonstrate a substantial rise. There were no significant changes in dry weight, blood pressure, Kt/V, or metabolic variables except for intradialytic hypotension. According to a meta-analysis, IDE raises Kt/V and maximum oxygen consumption during physical activity, reduces depression, and enhances the physical component of quality of life (QoL). SBP and DBP could both be dramatically reduced with IDE. In the end, IDE had no effect on the mental component of QoL. The enhanced muscle blood flow and expanded capillary surface area caused by IDE, on the other hand, may help HD remove toxins more effectively. There was also less dropout and increased compliance with the IDE [94] in addition to better acceptance and adherence.

10. Analyses of intradialytic vs. non-clinical exercise programmes

Home-based exercise (HBE) was found to be as effective as centre-based training in CKD patients who were not on dialysis. After 12 and 24 weeks, all of the cardiopulmonary metrics, including VO2peak, improved significantly. This was also seen during follow-up with respect to functional ability assessments. QoL and sleep both improved significantly [95].

In other research, researchers have compared the effects of IDE and HBE on the symptoms of HD. Neither their 6-minute walk test distance nor their pulse wave velocity changed significantly during the course of the study's 6-month follow-up period (which included blood pressure readings from both the peripheral and central nervous systems as well as physical activity). The second trial found that both groups' levels of physical activity grew significantly over time. While the one-legged standing test had a significant group-time interaction, the Short Physical Performance Battery, the timed up-and-go test, the STS-10 right and left hand grab, and the one-heel left leg rise all had a significant time influence. There was no change in the HRQoL score. Physical activity levels and physical function changed similarly in response to both treatments [96]. As a result, the effectiveness of IDE and HBE is comparable, and both produce positive effects.

11. Serum phosphate levels in a group of haemodialysis patients

Hyperphosphatemia, one of the comorbidities commonly associated with increased cardiovascular risk, is caused by reduced renal excretion of phosphate in CKD patients. Reduced hyperphosphatemia reduces the risk of vascular calcification in patients on pre-dialysis and MHD therapy. Medical intervention (active vitamin D, phosphate chelators, and calcimimetics) and diet are crucial in the treatment of mineral bone disorder-CKD. PA affects phosphate absorption in the gut.

According to a study, active HD patients had the highest levels of serum phosphate, and the link between the two was determined to be direct. The levels of serum phosphate were shown to be closely linked to those of serum calcium and albumin. An unanticipated rise in serum phosphate levels should be minimised and overall results should be improved by tailoring nutritional advice for chronic HD patients according to their amount of physical activity [97].

Patients who were hyperphosphatemic at baseline, but not the general population, did not improve appreciably following a 12-month moderate-intensity aerobic IDE, according to the results of another trial. The malnourished inflammation score remained constant throughout the study. A small but statistically insignificant rise in the QoL visual analogue scale was associated with IDE. Patients with hyperphosphatemia benefited the most from 45 minutes of aerobic IDE, which was reported to be both safe and effective [98].

Cycling on stationary cycles while getting haemodialysis was found to be a safe and helpful therapeutic intervention for individuals with end-stage renal disease in a recent RCT (ESRD). After an 8-week intervention, serum phosphate and parathyroid hormone levels improved dramatically, whereas albumin and calcium levels remained stable [99].

12. Conclusion

Sedentary lifestyles and lack of regular physical activity are common among CKD patients. This way of living has a negative impact on HRQoL and raises the risk of disease and death. Physical activity enhances physiological, functional, quality of life (QoL), and psychological components when done on a regular basis. When used in conjunction with dialysis, it improves both efficiency and adherence. However, overcoming the obstacle to regular PE and prescribing personalised PPE to CKD patients should be prioritised.

Author details

Dhanya Michael[1*], Joseph S. Fidelis[2] and Sijo Joseph Pakalomattom[3]

1 Lourdes Post Graduate Institute of Medical Sciences and Research, Kochi, Kerala, India

2 Critical Care Consultant Annai Velankanni Nursing Home Murugankurchi, Palayamkottai, Tirunelveli, Tamil Nadu, India

3 Government Medical College, Ernakulum, Kerala, India

*Address all correspondence to: dhanyamichaelmay9@gmail.com

References

[1] Thaniyath TA. The quality of life of the patients under palliative care: The features of appropriate assessment tools and the impact of early integration of palliative care. Palliative Care. 2019. DOI: 10.5772/intechopen.85161

[2] Liao PS. Perceived quality of life. In: Michalos AC, editor. Encyclopedia of Quality of Life and Well-Being Research. Dordrecht: Springer; 2014. DOI: 10.1007/978-94-007-0753-5_2129

[3] Hand C. Measuring health-related quality of life in adults with chronic conditions in primary care settings: Critical review of concepts and 3 tools [Mesurer la qualité de vie liée à la santé des adultes souffrant de problèmes chroniques en milieux de soins primaires]. Canadian Family Physician. 2016;**62**(7):e375-e383

[4] Parrish AR. Advances in chronic kidney disease. International Journal of Molecular Sciences. 2016;**17**(8):1314. DOI: 10.3390/ijms17081314

[5] Jeloka TK, Upase S, Chitikeshi S. Monthly cost of three sessions a day peritoneal dialysis is same as of thrice a week hemodialysis in self-paying Indian patients. Indian Journal of Nephrology. 2012;**22**:39-41

[6] Ahlawat R, Tiwari P, D'Cruz S. Direct cost for treating chronic kidney disease at an outpatient setting of a tertiary hospital: Evidence from a cross-sectional study. Value in Health Regional Issues. 2017;**12**:36-40. DOI: 10.1016/j.vhri.2016.10.003

[7] Pei M, Aguiar R, Pagels AA, Heimbürger O, Stenvinkel P, Bárány P, et al. Health-related quality of life as predictor of mortality in end-stage renal disease patients: an observational study. BMC Nephrology. 2019;**20**:144. DOI: 10.1186/s12882-019-1318-x

[8] Mapes DL, Lopes AA, Satayathum S, McCullough KP, Goodkin DA, Locatelli F, et al. Health-related quality of life as a predictor of mortality and hospitalization: the Dialysis Outcomes and Practice Patterns Study (DOPPS). Kidney International. 2003;**64**(1): 339-349. DOI: 10.1046/j.1523-1755.2003.00072.x

[9] Yamagata K, Hoshino J, Sugiyama H, Hanafusa N, Shibagaki Y, Komatsu Y, et al. Clinical practice guideline for renal rehabilitation: systematic reviews and recommendations of exercise therapies in patients with kidney diseases. Renal Replacement Therapy. 2019;**5**:28. DOI: 10.1186/s41100-019-0209-8

[10] Mallamaci F, Pisano A, Tripepi G. Physical activity in chronic kidney disease and the EXerCise Introduction To Enhance trial. Nephrology, Dialysis, Transplantation. 2020;**35**(Supplement_2):ii18-ii22. DOI: 10.1093/ndt/gfaa012

[11] World Health Organization. Global Recommendations on Physical Activity for Health. Geneva: WHO Press; 2010 Available from: https://www.who.int/dietphysicalactivity/global-PA-recs-2010.pdf [Accessed: 23 August 2021]

[12] Burkhalter TM, Hillman CH. A narrative review of physical activity, nutrition, and obesity to cognition and scholastic performance across the human lifespan. Advances in Nutrition: An International Review Journal. 2011;**2**:201S-206S. DOI: 10.3945/an.111.000331

[13] Amaral LSB, Souza CS, Lima HN, Soares TJ. Influence of exercise training on diabetic kidney disease: A brief physiological approach. Experimental Biology and Medicine (Maywood, N.J.). 2020;**245**(13):1142-1154. DOI: 10.1177/1535370220928986

[14] Heiwe S, Jacobson SH. Exercise training for adults with chronic kidney disease. Cochrane Database of Systematic Reviews. 2011;**10**:Cd003236

[15] Lobo C, Neyra-Bohorquez PP, Seco-Calvo J. Aerobic exercise effects in renal function and quality of life of patients with advanced chronic kidney disease. Rev Assoc Med Bras. 2019;**65**(5):657-662. DOI: 10.1590/1806-9282.65.5.657

[16] Mohammed MF, Draz AH, Karkousha RN, El-Nahas NG. Effect of aerobic exercises on functional capacity in patients under hemodialysis. The Medical Journal of Cairo University. 2019;**87**(7):4077-4085

[17] Mohseni R, Emami Zeydi A, Ilali E, Adib-Hajbaghery M, Makhlough A. The effect of intradialytic aerobic exercise on dialysis efficacy in hemodialysis patients: a randomized controlled trial. Oman Medical Journal. 2013;**28**(5): 345-349. DOI: 10.5001/omj.2013.99

[18] Frih B, Jaafar H, Mkacher W, Ben Salah Z, Hammami M, Frih A. The effect of interdialytic combined resistance and aerobic exercise training on health related outcomes in chronic hemodialysis patients: The Tunisian randomized controlled study. Frontiers in Physiology. 2017;**8**:288. DOI: 10.3389/fphys.2017.00288

[19] Abd-Elmonem AM, Al-Tohamy AM, Galal RE, Abd-Elhalim FA. Effects of progressive resistance exercises on quality of life and functional capacity in pediatric patients with chronic kidney disease: A randomized trail. Journal of Musculoskeletal & Neuronal Interactions. 2019;**19**(2):187-195

[20] Hoshino J. Renal rehabilitation: Exercise intervention and nutritional support in dialysis patients. Nutrients. 2021;**13**:1444. DOI: 10.3390/nu13051444

[21] Manfredini F, Mallamaci F, Catizone L, Zoccali C. The burden of physical inactivity in chronic kidney disease: is there an exit strategy? Nephrology, Dialysis, Transplantation. 2012;**27**(6):2143-2145. DOI: 10.1093/ndt/gfs120

[22] Arija V, Villalobos F, Pedret R, Vinuesa A, Jovani D, Pascual G, et al. Physical activity, cardiovascular health, quality of life and blood pressure control in hypertensive subjects: randomized clinical trial. Health and Quality of Life Outcomes. 2018;**16**(1):184-194

[23] Cao RY, Zheng H, Mi Q, Li Q, Yuan W, Ding Y, et al. Aerobic exercise-based cardiac rehabilitation in Chinese patients with coronary heart disease: study protocol for a pilot randomized controlled trial. Trials. 2018;**19**(1): 363-369

[24] Howden EJ, Leano R, Petchey W, Coombes JS, Isbel NM, Marwick TH. Effects of exercise and lifestyle intervention on cardiovascular function in CKD. Clinical Journal of the American Society of Nephrology. 2013;**8**(9):1494-1501

[25] Anderson E, Durstine JL. Physical activity, exercise, and chronic diseases: A brief review. SMHS. 2019;**1**(1):3-10. DOI: 10.1016/j.smhs.2019.08.006

[26] Nakamura K, Sasaki T, Yamamoto S, Hayashi H, Ako S, Tanaka Y. Effects of exercise on kidney and physical function in patients with non-dialysis chronic kidney disease: a systematic review and meta-analysis. Scientific Reports. 2020;**10**:18195. DOI: 10.1038/s41598-020-75405-x

[27] MacKinnon HJ et al. The association of physical function and physical activity with all-cause mortality and adverse clinical outcomes in nondialysis chronic kidney disease: A systematic review. Therapeutic Advances in Chronic Disease. 2018;**9**(11):209-226. DOI: 10.1177/2040622318785575

[28] Ghafourifard M, Mehrizade B, Hassankhani H, Heidari M. Hemodialysis patients perceived exercise benefits and barriers: the association with health-related quality of life. BMC Nephrology. 2021;**22**:94. DOI: 10.1186/s12882-021-02292-3

[29] Filipcic T, Bogataj S, Pajek J, Pajek M. Physical activity and quality of life in hemodialysis patients and healthy controls: A cross-sectional study. International Journal of Environmental Research and Public Health. 2021;**18**:1978. DOI: 10.3390/ijerph18041978

[30] Pinckard K, Baskin KK, Stanford KI. Effects of exercise to improve cardiovascular health. Frontiers in Cardiovascular Medicine. 2019;**6**:69. DOI: 10.3389/fcvm.2019.00069

[31] Nystoriak MA, Bhatnagar A. Cardiovascular effects and benefits of exercise. Frontiers in Cardiovascular Medicine. 2018;**5**:135. DOI: 10.3389/fcvm.2018.00135

[32] Helmrich SP, Ragland DR, Leung RW, et al. Physical activity and reduced occurrence of non-insulin-dependent diabetes mellitus. The New England Journal of Medicine. 1991;**325**: 147-152. DOI: 10.1056/NEJM199107183250302

[33] Distefano G, Goodpaster BH. Effects of exercise and aging on skeletal muscle. Cold Spring Harbor Perspectives in Medicine. 2018;**8**(3):a029785. DOI: 10.1101/cshperspect.a029785

[34] Mandolesi L, Polverino A, Montuori S, Foti F, Ferraioli G, Sorrentino P, et al. Effects of physical exercise on cognitive functioning and wellbeing: Biological and psychological benefits. Frontiers in Psychology. 2018;**9**:509. DOI: 10.3389/fpsyg.2018.00509

[35] Penedo FJ, Dahn JR. Exercise and well-being: A review of mental and physical health benefits associated with physical activity. Current Opinion in Psychiatry. 2005;**18**(2):189-193. DOI: 10.1097/00001504-200503000-00013

[36] Kujala UM. Benefits of exercise therapy for chronic diseases. British Journal of Sports Medicine. 2006;**40**(1):3-4. DOI: 10.1136/bjsm.2005.021717

[37] Warburton DE, Nicol CW, Bredin SS. Health benefits of physical activity: The evidence. CMAJ. 2006;**174**(6):801-809. DOI: 10.1503/cmaj.051351

[38] Reiner M, Niermann C, Jekauc D, Woll A. Long-term health benefits of physical activity – a systematic review of longitudinal studies. BMC Public Health. 2013;**13**:813. DOI: 10.1186/1471-2458-13-813

[39] Qiu Z, Zheng K, Zhang H, Feng J, Wang L, Zhou H. Physical exercise and patients with chronic renal failure: A meta-analysis. BioMed Research International. 2017;**2017**(7191826):8. DOI: 10.1155/2017/7191826

[40] Manfredini F, Mallamaci F, D'Arrigo G, et al. Exercise in patients on dialysis: A multicenter, randomized clinical trial. Journal of the American Society of Nephrology. 2017;**28**:1259-1268

[41] Zhang L, Wang Y, Xiong L, Luo Y, Huang Z, Yi B. Exercise therapy improves eGFR, and reduces blood pressure and BMI in non-dialysis CKD patients: evidence from a meta-analysis. BMC Nephrology. 2019;**20**:398. DOI: 10.1186/s12882-019-1586-5

[42] Anding K, Bar T, Trojniak-Hennig J, Kuchinke S, Krause R, Rost JM, et al. A structured exercise programme during haemodialysis for patients with chronic kidney disease: clinical benefit and

long-term adherence. BMJ Open. 2015;**5**:e008709. DOI: 10.1136/bmjopen-2015- 008709

[43] Huang M, Lv A, Wang J, Xu N, Ma G, Zhai Z, et al. Exercise training and outcomes in hemodialysis patients: Systematic review and meta-analysis. American Journal of Nephrology. 2019;**50**(4):240-254. DOI: 10.1159/000502447

[44] Chen SS, Al Mawed S, Unruh M. Health-related quality of life in end-stage renal disease patients: How often should we ask and what do we do with the answer? Blood Purification. 2016;**41**(1-3):218-224. DOI: 10.1159/000441462

[45] Joshi VD. Quality of life in end stage renal disease patients. World Journal of Nephrology. 2014;**3**(4):308-316. DOI: 10.5527/wjn.v3.i4.308

[46] Grubbs V, Tuot DS, Powe NR, O'Donoghue D, Chesla CA. System-level barriers and facilitators for foregoing or withdrawing dialysis: a qualitative study of nephrologists in the United States and England. American Journal of Kidney Diseases. 2017;**70**:602-610. DOI: 10.1053/j.ajkd.2016.12.015

[47] Cohen SD, Norris L, Acquaviva K, Peterson RA, Kimmel PL. Screening, diagnosis, and treatment of depression in patients with end-stage renal disease. Clinical Journal of the American Society of Nephrology. 2007;**2**:1332-1342. DOI: 10.2215/CJN.03951106

[48] Hedayati SS, Bosworth HB, Briley LP, et al. Death or hospitalization of patients on chronic hemodialysis is associated with a physician-based diagnosis of depression. Kidney International. 2008;**74**:930-936. DOI: 10.1038/ki.2008.311

[49] Sohn BK, Oh YK, Choi JS, et al. Effectiveness of group cognitive behavioral therapy with mindfulness in end-stage renal disease hemodialysis patients. Kidney Research and Clinical Practice. 2018;**37**:77-84. DOI: 10.23876/j.krcp.2018.37.1.77

[50] Kopple JD, Kim JC, Shapiro BB, et al. Factors affecting daily physical activity and physical performance in maintenance dialysis patients. Journal of Renal Nutrition. 2015;**25**:217-222. DOI: 10.1053/j.jrn.2014.10.017

[51] Findlay MD, Mark PB. Reduced and declining physical function in prevalent dialysis patients-identifying the vulnerable. Age and Ageing. 2017;**46**: 541-543. DOI: 10.1093/ageing/afx049

[52] Lee J, Kim YC, Kwon S, Li L, Oh S, Kim DH, et al. Impact of health-related quality of life on survival after dialysis initiation: A prospective cohort study in Korea. Kidney Research and Clinical Practice. 2020;**39**(4):426-440. DOI: 10.23876/j.krcp.20.065

[53] Tentori F, Elder SJ, Thumma J, Pisoni RL, Bommer J, Fissell RB, et al. Physical exercise among participants in the Dialysis Outcomes and Practice Patterns Study (DOPPS): Correlates and associated outcomes. Nephrology, Dialysis, Transplantation. 2010;**25**: 3050-3062

[54] Matsuzawa R, Matsunaga A, Wang G, Kutsuna T, Ishii A, Abe Y, et al. Habitual physical activity measured by accelerometer and survival in maintenance hemodialysis patients. Clinical Journal of the American Society of Nephrology. 2012;7:2010-2016

[55] Abdel-Kader K, Unruh ML, Weisbord SD. Symptom burden, depression, and quality of life in chronic and end-stage kidney disease. Clinical Journal of the American Society of Nephrology. 2009;**4**:1057-1064

[56] Robinson-Cohen C, Littman AJ, Duncan GE, Roshanravan B, Ikizler TA, Himmelfarb J, et al. Assessment of

physical activity in chronic kidney disease. Journal of Renal Nutrition. 2013;**23**:123-131. DOI: 10.1053/j.jrn.2012.04.008

[57] Makhlough A, Ilali E, Mohsen R, Shahmohammadi S. Effect of intradialytic aerobic exercise on serum electrolytes levels in hemodialysis patients. Iranian Journal of Kidney Diseases. 2012;**6**(2):119-123

[58] Kouidi E, Albani M, Natsis K, et al. The effects of exercise training on muscle atrophy in haemodialysis Patients. Nephrology, Dialysis, Transplantation. 1998;**13**:685-699

[59] Kirkman DL, Mullins P, Junglee NA, et al. Anabolic exercise in haemodialysis patients: a randomised controlled pilot study. Journal of Cachexia, Sarcopenia and Muscle. 2014;**5**:199-207

[60] Hood DA, Memme JM, Oliveira AN, et al. Maintenance of skeletal muscle mitochondria in health, exercise, and aging. Annual Review of Physiology. 2019;**81**:19-41

[61] Heiwe S, Jacobson SH. Exercise training in adults with CKD: a systematic review and meta-analysis. American Journal of Kidney Diseases. 2014;**64**(3):383-393

[62] Lu Y, Wang Y, Lu Q. Effects of exercise on muscle fitness in dialysis patients: A systematic review and meta-analysis. American Journal of Nephrology. 2019;**50**:291-302. DOI: 10.1159/000502635

[63] Deligiannis A, D'Alessandro C, Cupisti A. Exercise training in dialysis patients: Impact on cardiovascular and skeletal muscle health. Clinical Kidney Journal. 2021;**14**(Supplement_2): ii25-ii33. DOI: 10.1093/ckj/sfaa273

[64] Deligiannis A, Kouidi E, Tassoulas E, et al. Cardiac effects of exercise rehabilitation in hemodialysis patients. International Journal of Cardiology. 1999;**70**:253-266

[65] Momeni A, Nematolahi A, Nasr M. Effect of intradialytic exercise on echocardiographic findings in hemodialysis patients. Iranian Journal of Kidney Diseases. 2014;**8**:207-211

[66] Parsons TL, Toffelmire EB, King-VanVlack CE. The effect of an exercise program during hemodialysis on dialysis efficacy, blood pressure and quality of life in end-stage renal disease (ESRD) patients. Clinical Nephrology. 2004;**61**:261-274

[67] Mustata S, Chan C, Lai V, Miller JA. Impact of an exercise program on arterial stiffness and insulin resistance in hemodialysis patients. Journal of the American Society of Nephrology. 2004;**15**(10):2713-2718. DOI: 10.1097/01.ASN.0000140256.21892.89

[68] Houmard JA, Tanner CJ, Slentz CA, Duscha BD, McCartney JS, Kraus WE. The effect of the volume and intensity of exercise training on insulin sensitivity. Journal of Applied Physiology. 2004;**96**:101-106

[69] Toyama K, Sugiyama S, Oka H, Sumida H, Ogawa H. Exercise therapy correlates with improving renal function through modifying lipid metabolism in patients with cardiovascular disease and chronic kidney disease. Journal of Cardiology. 2010;**56**(2):142-146. DOI: 10.1016/j.jjcc.2010.06.007

[70] Greenwood SA, Koufaki P, Mercer TH, MacLaughlin HL, Rush R, Lindup H, et al. Effect of exercise training on estimated GFR, vascular health, and cardiorespiratory fitness in patients with CKD: A pilot randomized controlled trial. American Journal of Kidney Diseases. 2015;**65**(3):425-434. DOI: 10.1053/j.ajkd.2014.07.015

[71] Hiraki K, Shibagaki Y, Izawa KP, Hotta C, Wakamiya A, Sakurada T, et al.

Effects of home-based exercise on predialysis chronic kidney disease patients: A randomized pilot and feasibility trial. BMC Nephrology. 2017;**18**:198

[72] de Olival FA, Alves dos Santos Sens Y, Bertoni Xavier V, Antonio Miorin L, dos Santos Alves VL. Functional and respiratory capacity of patients with chronic kidney disease undergoing cycle ergometer training during hemodialysis sessions: a randomized clinical trial. International Journal of Nephrology. 2019;**2019**:7857824

[73] Thiebaud RS, Funk MD, Abe T. Home-based resistance training for older adults: a systematic review. Geriatrics & Gerontology International. 2014;**14**:750-757

[74] Myers J, Chan K, Chen Y, Lit Y, Patti A, Massaband P, et al. Effect of a home-based exercise program on indices of physical function and quality of life in elderly maintenance hemodialysis patients. Kidney & Blood Pressure Research. 2021;**46**:196-206. DOI: 10.1159/000514269

[75] Kirkman DL, Lennon-Edwards S, Edwards DG. The importance of exercise for chronic kidney disease patients. Journal of Renal Nutrition. 2014;**24**(6):e51-e53

[76] Maddux DW, West C. The benefits of exercise for CKD patients. Nephrology News & Issues. 2012;**26**(12):44, 46, 48

[77] Aucella F, Valente GL, Catizone L. The role of physical activity in the CKD setting. Kidney & Blood Pressure Research. 2014;**39**:97-106. DOI: 10.1159/000355783

[78] Patel H, Alkhawam H, Madanieh R, Shah N, Kosmas CE, Vittorio TJ. Aerobic vs anaerobic exercise training effects on the cardiovascular system. World Journal of Cardiology. 2017;**9**(2): 134-138. DOI: 10.4330/wjc.v9.i2.134

[79] Lin X, Zhang X, Guo J, Roberts CK, McKenzie S, Wu WC, et al. Effects of exercise training on cardiorespiratory fitness and biomarkers of cardiometabolic health: A systematic review and meta-analysis of randomized controlled trials. Journal of the American Heart Association. 2015;**4**:e002014. DOI: 10.1161/JAHA.115.002014

[80] Kosmadakis GC, Bevington A, Smith AC, Clapp EL, Viana JL, Bishop NC, et al. Physical exercise in patients with severe kidney disease. Nephron. Clinical Practice. 2010;**115**: c7-c16. DOI: 10.1159/000286344

[81] Sietsema KE, Amato A, Adler SG, Brass EP. Exercise capacity as a predictor of survival among ambulatory patients with end-stage renal disease. Kidney International. 2004;**65**:719-724

[82] Evans RW, Manninen DL, Garrison LP Jr, Hart LG, Blagg CR, Gutman RA, et al. The quality of life of patients with end-stage renal disease. The New England Journal of Medicine. 1985;**312**:553-559

[83] Ossareh S, Roozbeh J, Krishnan M, Liakopoulos V, Bargman JM, Oreopoulos DG. Fatigue in chronic peritoneal dialysis patients. International Urology and Nephrology. 2003;**35**:535-541

[84] Canadian Erythropoietin Study Group. Association between recombinant human erythropoietin and quality of life and exercise capacity of patients receiving haemodialysis. BMJ. 1990;**300**:573-578

[85] Beusterien KM, Nissenson AR, Port FK, Kelly M, Steinwald B, Ware JE Jr. The effects of recombinant human erythropoietin on functional health and well-being in chronic dialysis patients.

Journal of the American Society of Nephrology. 1996;**7**:763-773

[86] Macdougall IC, Lewis NP, Saunders MJ, Cochlin DL, Davies ME, Hutton RD, et al. Long-term cardiorespiratory effects of amelioration of renal anaemia by erythropoietin. Lancet. 1990;**335**:489-493

[87] Johansen KL, Finkelstein FO, Revicki DA, Gitlin M, Evans C, Mayne TJ. Systematic review and meta-analysis of exercise tolerance and physical functioning in dialysis patients treated with erythropoiesis-stimulating agents. American Journal of Kidney Diseases. 2010;**55**:535-548

[88] Painter P, Moore G, Carlson L, Paul S, Myll J, Phillips W, et al. Effects of exercise training plus normalization of hematocrit on exercise capacity and health-related quality of life. American Journal of Kidney Diseases. 2002;**39**:257-265

[89] Painter PL, Nelson-Worel JN, Hill MM, Thornbery DR, Shelp WR, Harrington AR, et al. Effects of exercise training during hemodialysis. Nephron. 1986;**43**:87-92

[90] Goldberg AP, Geltman EM, Hagberg JM, Gavin JR 3rd, Delmez JA, Carney RM, et al. Therapeutic benefits of exercise training for hemodialysis patients. Kidney International. Supplement. 1983;**16**:S303-S309

[91] Moore GE, Parsons DB, Stray-Gundersen J, Painter PL, Brinker KR, Mitchell JH. Uremic myopathy limits aerobic capacity in hemodialysis patients. American Journal of Kidney Diseases. 1993;**22**:277-287

[92] Dobre M, Meyer TW, Hostetter TH. Searching for uremic toxins. Clinical Journal of the American Society of Nephrology. 2013;**8**:322-327

[93] Stray-Gundersen J, Howden EJ, Parsons DB, Thompson JR. Neither hematocrit normalization nor exercise training restores oxygen consumption to normal levels in hemodialysis patients. Journal of the American Society of Nephrology. 2016;**27**(12):3769-3779. DOI: 10.1681/ASN.2015091034

[94] Rhee SY, Song JK, Hong SC, Choi JW, Jeon HJ, Shin DH, et al. Intradialytic exercise improves physical function and reduces intradialytic hypotension and depression in hemodialysis patients. The Korean Journal of Internal Medicine. 2019;**34**(3):588-598. DOI: 10.3904/kjim.2017.020

[95] Aoike DT, Baria F, Kamimura MA, Ammirati A, Cuppari L. Home-based versus center-based aerobic exercise on cardiopulmonary performance, physical function, quality of life and quality of sleep of overweight patients with chronic kidney disease. Clinical and Experimental Nephrology. 2018;**22**:87-98. DOI: 10.1007/s10157-017-1429-2

[96] Ortega-Pérez de Villar L, Martínez-Olmos FJ, de Borja P-DF, Benavent-Caballer V, Montañez-Aguilera FJ, Mercer T, et al. Comparison of intradialytic versus home-based exercise programs on physical functioning, physical activity level, adherence, and health-related quality of life: pilot study. Scientific Reports. 2020;**10**:8302. DOI: 10.1038/s41598-020-64372-y

[97] Stroescu AEB, Peride I, Constantin AM, David C, Sinescu RD, Niculae A. The influence of physical activity on serum phosphate levels in a group of hemodialysis patients. Revista de Chimie. 2017;**68**(7):1581-1585. DOI: 10.37358/RC.17.7.5721

[98] Salhab N, Alrukhaimi M, Kooman J, et al. Effect of intradialytic exercise on hyperphosphatemia and malnutrition. Nutrients. 2019;**11**(10):2464. DOI: 10.3390/nu11102464

[99] Dashtidehkordi A, Shahgholian N, Sadeghian J. The effect of Exercise during hemodialysis on serum levels of Albumin, calcium, phosphorus and parathyroid hormone: a randomized clinical trial. Res Sq. 2018;**68**(7):1581-1585. DOI: 10.21203/rs.3.rs-446114/v1

Chapter 2

The Hope of Patients Undergoing Hemodialysis and Peritoneal Dialysis

Rayane Alves Moreira, Moema da Silva Borges and Ana Luiza Gonçalves Moura

Abstract

Hope facilitates the adaptation of disability to health care. In the context of chronic kidney disease, hope is a relevant factor, as it encourages patients to adhere to treatments that include invasive procedures, change their lifestyle, and remain, even if weakened, in a painful and delicate treatment. Currently, there are three main therapies for the advanced stage of chronic kidney disease: hemodialysis (HD), peritoneal dialysis (PD), and kidney transplantation. The last is the ideal treatment, but not all patients can be transplanted, for different reasons. Thus, most individuals in a situation of renal failure undergo hemodialysis or peritoneal dialysis. Kidney failure is an unpleasant and difficult disease to accept. In general, a chronic renal patient on dialysis can live in anguish, fear, and insecurity about their subsequent quality of life. Thus, you can abandon your everyday life desires as well as your dreams of enjoying more favorable conditions in the future. The Herth Hope Scale aims to quantify hope in individuals in clinical situations. Therefore, this chapter will deal with the level of hope of dialysis patients, proposing a comparison between those who undergo hemodialysis and peritoneal dialysis.

Keywords: hope, chronic kidney disease, nursing, renal dialysis, kidney transplantation

1. Introduction

Hope is a construct that helps to adapt to the treatment of various diseases [1]. It is a multidimensional, universal, and dynamic concept, being described as a cognitive process through which individuals actively pursue their goals, in an effort to move from the current situation toward new, more favorable conditions in the future [2].

This multidimensional concept allows the feeling of hope to permeate different disciplines. Because it has many approaches, it reveals itself as a transversal phenomenon, with multiple meanings, covering different areas of knowledge [3]. It is an individualized and subjective feeling, lived in a unique and personal way.

In the health area, hope is a concept that has gained increasing importance, especially for nurses who have a fundamental role in health promotion, as they are professionals who are in a privileged position to favor this feeling for those who receive their care [4].

In the context of chronic kidney disease (CKD), hope is a relevant factor, as it is what leads the patient to undergo relentless invasive procedures to change their lifestyle and to remain, even if weakened, in painful and delicate treatment [5].

According to data from the "Brazilian Chronic Dialysis Survey," in 2019, there were about 139,691,000 patients with dialysis in Brazil [6]. These patients face severe limitations, especially physical and emotional, imposed by hemodialysis and/or peritoneal dialysis [7, 8].

The growing interest in the concept of hope in professional health areas reflects the commitment and concern to reinforce this aspect with patients, in order to contribute to training to deal with situations of crisis and suffering [9].

Thus, given the alarming statistics and so many challenges faced by chronic kidney patients, whether in the physical, mental, social, or spiritual sphere, it is important to analyze the level of hope of patients with chronic kidney disease, due to its relevance in the patient's adaptation to treatment.

2. Hope in the health area

Hope is a multidimensional, universal, and dynamic concept. It can be described as a cognitive process through which people actively pursue their goals, in an effort to move out of a current situation, toward new, more favorable conditions in the future [2]. It is a construct that facilitates the adaptation of individuals to different health treatments [1]. In view of this, as it is associated with this concept, hope does not belong to a single discipline, it manifests itself as a transversal phenomenon, with multiple meanings, covering different areas of knowledge [3].

In the field of health, hope has become of paramount importance, gaining more and more relevance and strength. Thus, in the field of nursing, nurses occupy a privileged position to encourage this feeling with patients who receive their care [4]. Therefore, it is necessary that these professionals understand that hope allows their patients' personal, clinical, and social adaptive efforts to be successful, in order to enable a possible intervention through actions, aiming to help their patients to adapt to a life reconstructed and modified [1].

In this context, in the face of kidney diseases, hope is a relevant factor [5]. CKD is an unpleasant and difficult disease to accept. Patients with CKD are individuals who face severe limitations, especially physical and emotional, imposed by hemodialysis and/or peritoneal dialysis, at the risk of living in anguish, fear, and deep uncertainty about their future, giving up their daily desires for life, and their dreams of having a pleasant future [7, 8, 10].

In summary, it can be said that the limitations resulting from kidney diseases produce negative effects on the energy and vitality levels of patients, as they establish restrictions related to common daily activities, causing severe changes in productive and personal life, which can lead to a functional disability of the individual [7, 11]. Given the above, identifying the level of hope of CKD patients can contribute to better coping with the treatment and the limitations/restrictions it imposes, preparing them to deal resiliently with the pain of the moment and the uncertainties of the future [5, 12].

2.1 The feeling of hope

Studies have shown that the induction of the state of hope expands the human being's field of attention, develop positive emotions, intuition, and creativity [13] that favor the release of hormones that alter the body system, favoring positive thoughts and emotions [14].

Therefore, positive emotions promote mental and physical health, as these feelings reinforce resilience in the face of adversity, increase happiness, and favor psychological growth [13].

Hope is a part of positive emotions, along with love, joy, forgiveness, compassion, faith, reverence, enthusiasm, contentment, satisfaction, a sense of control, and gratitude. Hope is a feeling that leads to emotions, capable of providing well-being and improving the quality of life of individuals, especially those undergoing treatment for chronic and/or severe diseases [15]. Positive emotions connect us with our experience of the divine; however, we conceive of it. In this way, spirituality works as a kind of amalgamation of positive emotions [16].

In this line of argument, it can be said that hope is not a mere cognitive defense mechanism, but a positive emotion. According to Vaillant, [16] the feeling of hope allows us to deal with reality in a lucid way and look death directly in the eyes and accept the reality of incurable diseases. Paradoxically, the greater the suffering, the greater the power of honest hope, as the individual embraces the truth.

The opposite of hope is hopelessness (or despair), which is reflected in our organism through negative emotions that cause metabolic and cardiac excitement, activated by the sympathetic autonomic nervous system, triggering reactions such as fight or flight. Negative emotions, such as fear and anger, limit the individual's attention, causing him/her to become entangled in unnecessary detail without seeing the context. So, suffering is hope destroyed, and it causes pain, loss of self-control, and despair. However, if the end of hope turns pain into suffering, the return of hope makes suffering a tolerable pain. Suffering is the loss of autonomy, and hope is your restoration of personal power and self-confidence [16].

Similarly, the opposite of trust is distrust, and the opposite of hope is despair. Without trust, we are cautious and even paranoid. Hopeless, we are completely depressed. Hopelessness and clinical depression are the same thing and can be fatal. Soon, hope will be born out of an involuntary need to function effectively in the face of threatening situations. It is a source of comforting emotion and reminds us that tomorrow can always be better. Hope and despair are feelings, and true hope has its roots in the heart, music, and cognitive awareness [16].

Hope is born from the dialectic of feelings of indignation and anger. The indignation lies in the refusal to live in a situation of misery (or inequity) that prevents human beings from going beyond, from being more. Anger and indignation are motivating feelings of denial and make the individual look for changes in an undesirable situation. Ultimately, hope is a feeling capable of transforming reality, of making human beings always seek their best [17].

Added to this, hope must be distinguished from desire, since the latter is associated with words and the left side of the brain. On the other hand, hope is made up of images and relates to the right side of the brain. Desiring something is effortless. Hope, in fact, takes a lot of effort and shapes real life. It reflects our ability to imagine a positive and realistic future. Hope is then emotional, energizing, and it gives strength. Desire, in turn, is a passive, cognitive feeling and can be debilitating [16].

Furthermore, in the context of health, hope leads the patient to take the focus off the pain. Hope is the result of our first experience with zeal, it comes from the visceral feeling, not from a cognitive knowledge that we are important and that we will win someday [16].

2.2 The hope of the chronic kidney patient

In the context of kidney diseases, available treatments such as hemodialysis (HD), peritoneal dialysis (PD), and kidney transplantation have profound implications, both physical and emotional [18]. It is known that renal replacement therapies (RRT) have increased the survival of patients with chronic kidney disease (CKD), but it is important to emphasize that they generate negative impacts on these people's lives [19].

Soon, nursing care, which in its essence seeks integrality of action, defined by a singular objective according to the particular need of each individual, considers human needs, in the physical, emotional, mental, and spiritual dimensions, aiming to promote the feeling of hope [20].

In the clinical management of CKD, the nursing team knows the importance of maintaining the feeling of hope, as the treatment generates frustration and limitations, due to various restrictions, such as maintaining a specific diet associated with water restrictions and changes in body appearance in the reason for the presence of the catheter for vascular access or the arteriovenous fistula. Thus, the patient lives daily with an incurable disease, associated with a long-lasting painful treatment, with possible complications, generating even greater limitations and changes of great impact [21].

Dialysis has negative effects on individuals' energy and vitality levels. The various restrictions related to daily activities and the severe changes in productive and personal life can lead to functional disability [7, 11, 18].

Chronic kidney patients face a drastic transformation in their daily lives, experiencing various limitations such as painful treatment, controlled diet, changes in family life, changes in professional and social life [22]. In this sense, the new life condition of these individuals affects not only their physical condition but also their social, family, economic, psychological, and spiritual dimensions, due to the prolonged period of exposure to long and stressful situations, inherent to the therapeutic procedures of the renal syndrome [23].

It is a fact that dialysis therapy is essential, as there is no way to be different, as intervention is necessary. In this way, it symbolizes the breadth of their suffering, as it affects the patients' lives as a way of imprisoning their entire existential potential, in the face of a difficult, inflexible reality, full of necessary restrictions. However, a good level of hope echoes in their heart, the possibility of transplantation reminds them of a "light at the end of the tunnel," given the inspiration of having a "normal life," far from the limitations imposed by dialysis [20].

The psychosocial impact of a chronic disease, such as the end-stage of kidney injury, is intense and deserves attention as a stressor, as feelings of anger with the treatment and loss of stimulus to maintain balance are common, leading patients to miss the dialysis sessions, not respecting water restrictions, drinking alcoholic beverages, and even using drugs [11].

Kidney disease is unpleasant and difficult to accept. Chronic renal dialysis patients run the risk of living in anguish, fear, and deep uncertainty about the future, with a great possibility of abandoning their daily life pleasures, as well as their dreams of having a blessed future [10]. Thus, there may be the triggering of doubts about their life expectancy, in addition to fear and other negative feelings [23]. In this sense, suicidal thoughts, poor perception of health, and the lack of hope to improve their quality of life are common feelings throughout the process [22].

Therefore, it is expected that the patient will present feelings of hopelessness, given the huge impact that CKD causes, both in the individual's personal and professional life. In this situation, maintaining hope is a valuable process in the coping process [21].

The individuals with CKD in the disease process may lose autonomy, with a consequent reduction of hope in the continuity of their own life, since different forms of lifestyle interfere, which can interrupt or hinder their insertion in the means of production in society, dramatically affecting their daily life. Thus, the patients become dependent on constant and permanent care from the health service and a machine [24].

The illness process of the kidney patient is intensely experienced, associated with various manifestations of personal behavior, from the discovery of the disease to the possibility of kidney transplantation. Kidney transplantation is desired by most patients. The term "new kidney" represents a healthy kidney, hope for resuming life, independence from the machine, and the "cure" related to faith. Attachment to belief is mentioned by patients, as it brings comfort and hope, strengthening and promoting the well-being of CKD waiting for a new kidney [25].

The patient awaiting kidney transplantation experiences negative and positive feelings. Negative feelings consist of insecurity, uncertainty, lack of autonomy, dependence, fear, lack of clarity, high perspective, difficulty in coping, inner conflict, hopelessness, and nonconformity. The positive ones, on the other hand, constitute the hope of happiness, will to live, well-being, overcoming difficulties, desire to maintain life, and search for quality of life [20].

The transplant is expected in the time in which the patient's experience is lived, a time full of meanings. It is a time to be-wait. Time in which you learn to be attentive and prepared, to fulfill the meeting with an uncertain future that awaits you. An uncertain future that will arrive unexpectedly and unannounced, meaning the end of the suffering that has been experienced since the moment of CKD diagnosis. Therefore, the option for transplantation is the hope of improving quality of life [26].

Generally, transplant recipients are aware of the finitude of the kidney. The duration of the organ is a continuous issue that permeates the lives of transplant patients, as some factors can influence its duration, such as the body's defense against foreign agents and the emergence of new diseases. The challenge for transplant recipients is to ensure that the graft lasts as long as possible [26].

The transplant requires a lot of care, such as the use of various medications, and there are risks of complications, including death, if the donated kidney is rejected by the recipient's body [1, 27].

In a survey conducted in a hemodialysis clinic of a public hospital in Brasília, it can be seen the patients registered on the kidney transplantation waiting list (mostly young and of working age) had lower levels of hope than those who weren't, which suggests that patients who are not registered on the transplantation waiting list feel safe and adapted to hemodialysis [28].

Another research pointed out that although transplantation can be seen as a way of "liberation," patients know that it does not reflect the possibility of total rescue of the aspects of life left behind. In this sense, transplantation does not mean the total and definitive resolution of the "problems," since these individuals experienced an undesirable survival of quality of life, resulting from restrictions caused by CKD, as a sudden change in their daily lives, full of limitations, merciless treatment and with an inevitable thought of death. Thus, transplantation is seen as something new, with multiple meanings, limited by fear and disbelief [20].

In view of the COVID-19 pandemic scenario, potential deceased donors and actual kidney, heart, and cornea donors were significantly reduced. In addition to the SARS-CoV-2 being an impediment to organ donation, with the government measures of social isolation, the number of accidents decreased, thus impacting the brain deaths of possible donors [29].

Another aspect that contributes to the multiplicity of meanings is the awareness that the organ can fail at any time, feelings of anxiety and sadness, and the fear of losing the transplant and the consequence of returning to dialysis therapy. However, transplantation also promises to release the bonds imposed by the disease and treatment, allowing these individuals to make new plans and activities that the disease forced them to interrupt [26].

In summary, in the transplant phase, patients believe in success, due to the fact that it provides them with a lifestyle close to the "normality" experienced before the diagnosis of the disease. Kidney transplantation is associated with the life of a healthy individual, linked to the sense of being reborn and starting a new life. The new birth allows them to escape the space where they were confined by pain, suffering, and anguish [26].

Despite the ambiguity of feelings about the result of kidney transplantation, it is noted that transplantation fosters the feeling of hope of some individuals, who see in it an opportunity for a new life, with more freedom and quality. At the same time, it is a therapy that still causes fears and uncertainties regarding the success and duration of the procedure [27].

In this context, faith can be a source of hope, as it helps to deal with uncertainties in the transplant process, offering comfort and tranquility, being one of the most used coping strategies while waiting for the donation. Receiving a kidney donation is a way to free yourself [26].

Therefore, hope is beneficial to the health of these individuals, as it contributes to the empowerment of patients when dealing with crisis situations, aiming at maintaining the quality of life, setting goals, and promoting health [21].

There is no doubt that the events are reenacted, by encouraging the adherence of positive feelings, such as hope, for example, in order to enable the chronic renal patient on dialysis to face the disease optimistically, helping them to reestablish their health, so that they continue fighting for their survival. The hope in health recovery makes the patients travel long distances in search of the arduous treatment for their disease, such as the tireless invasive procedures, changes in their lifestyle, their routine, and even if weakened, they remain in treatment [5].

Without a doubt, hope can help them to position themselves in a positive way in the face of different situations in life.

Some scientific instruments aim to quantify hope in individuals in clinical situations, such as the Herth Hope Scale (EEH), developed by Herth (1992), originally called the Herth Hope Index [30].

The EEH is a scale that has 12 affirmative items. The grading of its items occurs using a four-point Likert-type scale: 4 indicates "completely agree" and 1 indicates "completely disagree." There are two – items 3 and 6 – that have inverted scores. The total score ranges from 12 to 48, and the higher the score, the higher the level of hope. It is a scale considered brief (it takes, on average, 10 minutes to complete) and easy to understand [9, 21].

The items on the EEH scale are composed of the following statements: (1) I am optimistic about life; (2) I have short-term and long-term plans; (3) I feel very lonely; (4) I can see possibilities in the midst of difficulties; (5) I have a faith that comforts me; (6) I am afraid of my future; (7) I can remember happy and pleasurable times; (8) I feel very strong; (9) I feel able to give and receive affection/love; (10) I know where I want to go; (11) I believe in the value of each day; (12) I feel that my life has value and usefulness.

The Herth Hope Scale is of great importance, as it is a validated instrument for the use of patients in clinical situations (chronic, oncological and/or palliative care patients, and family caregivers) and the planning of interventions in the scope of nursing services. Reliability was verified through internal consistency analysis represented by Cronbach's alpha coefficient of 0.834, which demonstrates a high reliability of the instrument [30].

In a research on the applicability of EEH in patients with chronic kidney disease, the result was obtained that despite all the limitations imposed by the treatment and by the disease itself, the studied population had a high level of hope. In these patients, it was observed that the item with the highest HSE score was that which refers to faith as a measure of comfort (item 5, "I have a faith that comforts me"). Therefore, it was possible to deduce that faith contributes to maintaining a high level of hope [28].

The same research compared the level of hope between patients undergoing hemodialysis and those undergoing peritoneal dialysis, there was no statistically significant difference, since both groups maintain a high level of hope, even with routine differences related to treatment [28].

The fact that motivated the comparison was the perspective that patients on peritoneal dialysis have a higher level of hope than those on hemodialysis, due to the fact that they dialyze at home and depend less on the modality. A study on the domain of self-care indicates that patients on peritoneal dialysis are favored because there is less loss in activities of daily living and more free time, causing minimal changes in their routine [31].

2.3 Treatment and nursing

The nursing team must plan care strategies for patients with CKD, with a view to increasing the patient's hope, seeking to minimize the aspects that impede adherence to treatment. A systematic review pointed out, through the analyzed studies, some strategies that should be implemented to survey the patient's needs, such as: listening to the patient/relatives, establishing an empathetic relationship and developing communication skills, maintaining a sense of humor, and encouraging positive memories; strengthen social/family support; strengthen spiritual support; explore patients' feelings; foster emotional and motivational strategies; discuss information about the disease; set realistic goals and encourage the person to look beyond the disease [32].

A study identified that young people have greater difficulty in adhering to treatment, due to issues involving immaturity and resistance to the restrictions imposed by the disease and hemodialysis itself. However, the nurses successfully managed the resistances encountered, favoring the acceptance of the disease and treatment, maintaining the spiritual connection and emotional balance at high through conversations with the young people, seeking during the appointments and clarifying doubts, fears, and insecurities [33].

By providing comprehensive care and due to prolonged contact with the patient, nurses are able to create an interpersonal relationship, which favors a therapeutic bond. In this way, the observation capacity is expanded, detecting verbal and non-verbal expressions indicative of relevant and contextual situations, which may or may not interact with the patient [20].

Nurses are essential agents for promoting hope. Thus, moments of conversation and interaction with patients are opportunities that encourage this feeling, according to the needs of each one. Although they also have their own personal, family, spiritual, and/or financial dilemmas and problems, nurses are professionals capable of positively interfering in the level of hope of patients with chronic kidney disease on dialysis, since, in their interventions, with light technologies, they deal with essential themes such as faith, beliefs, and religion [33].

Nursing teams must implement interventions aimed at promoting and maintaining hope strategies, favoring the planning of comprehensive care that aims to improve the quality of life of patients with CKD [33].

Therefore, it is important that the nursing team is aware of the complications of the disease, anxiety, and possible stresses that involve this condition. Thus, promoting and encouraging care, also through health education, is essential, with a view to reduce low self-esteem related to the evolution of treatment [34].

3. Conclusion

Despite all the limitations imposed by the disease, these patients still manage to maintain a good level of hope, supported by faith, religion, and a good support network.

Hope is a feeling that facilitates the adaptation to treatment and helps patients to support the limitations imposed by the disease. Thus, nursing is the profession that is closest to the patient in their hemodialysis routine, therefore, they must implement interventions aimed at promoting and maintaining hope strategies, favoring the planning of comprehensive care, aiming at a good quality of life.

Author details

Rayane Alves Moreira[1*], Moema da Silva Borges[1] and Ana Luiza Gonçalves Moura[2]

1 University of Brasilia, Brasilia, Brazil

2 Higher School of Health Sciences, Brasilia, Brazil

*Address all correspondence to: enfermeiraray@gmail.com

References

[1] Ferreira C, Guanilo MEE, Silva DMGV, Gonçalves N, Boell JEW, Mayer BLD. Evaluation of hope and resilience in people in hemodialytic treatment. Scientific Journal of Nursing at the University of Santa Maria. 2018;**8**(4):1-15

[2] Snyder CR. The Psychology of Hope: You Can Get There From Here. New York: Free Press; 1994

[3] Querido A. Hope as a focus of mental health nursing. Portuguese Journal of Mental Health Nursing. 2018;**6**:06-08

[4] Martins R, Domingues M, Andrade A, Cunha M, Martins C. Hope in hospitalized patients on continuous care units. Portuguese Journal of Mental Health Nursing. 2017;**5**:81-85

[5] Ottaviani AC, Souza EN, Drago NC, Mendiondo MSZ, Pavarini SCL, Orlandi FZ. Hope and spirituality among patients with chronic kidney disease undergoing hemodialysis: A correlational study. Latin American Journal of Nursing. 2014;**22**(2):248-254

[6] Neves P, Sesso R, Thomé F, Lugon J, Nasciento M. Brazilian dialysis survey 2019. Brazilian Journal of Nephrology. 2021;**43**(2):217-227

[7] Silva JCC, Paiva SSCP, Almeida RJ. Hemodialysis and its psychosocial impacts in childbearing age women. Santa Maria Journal. 2017;**43**(1):189-198

[8] Caveião C, Visentin A, Hey AP, Sales WB, Ferreira ML, Passos RL. Quality of life in women with chronic kidney disease submitted to hemodialysis. Health School Notebooks. 2017;**1**(11):20-33

[9] Herth K. Hope in the family caregiver of terminally ill people. National Library of Medicine. 1993;**18**(4):538-548

[10] Sales CA, Cassarotti MS, Piolli KC, Matsuda L. The feeling of hope in câncer patients: An existential analysis. Rene Journal. 2014;**15**(4):659-667

[11] Rudinicki T. Chronic renal patient: Experience of hemodialysis treatment. Journal Clinical Contexts. 2014;**7**(1): 105-116

[12] Schuster JT, Feldens V, Moehlecke BP, Ghislandi GM. Hope and depression in patients with câncer at a hospital in Southern Brazil. Scientific Journal Medical Association of Rio Grande do Sul. 2015;**59**(2):84-89

[13] Fredrickson BL, Losada MF. Positive affect and the complex dynamics of human flourishing. American Psychologist. 2005;**60**(5):678-686

[14] Wiedemann G, Pauli P, Dengler W, Lutenberger W, Birbaumer N, Buchkremer G. Frontal brain asymmetry as a biological substrate of emotions in patients with panic disorders. Archives of General Psychiatry. 1999;**56**(1):78-84

[15] Martins RML, Mestre MA. Hope and quality of life in the elderly. Millenium Journal. 2014;**47**:153-162

[16] Vaillant GE. Faith: Scientific Evidence. 1st ed. Barueri, São Paulo, Brasil: Manole; 2010

[17] Oliveira CT, Rodrigues VHG. Theoretical dialogues between Paulo Freire and Ernst Bloch: dialogues about the Principle and Pedagogy of Hope. Education: Theory & Practic. 2014;**24**(46):40-54

[18] Oller G, Ribeiro RCHM, Travagim DAS, Batista MA, Marques S, Kusumota L. Functional independence in patients with chronic kidney disease being treated with haemodialysis. Latin American Journal of Nursing. 2012; **20**(6):[08 screens]

[19] Gomes NDB, Leal NPR, Pimenta CJL, Martins KP, Ferreira GRS, Costa KNFMC. Quality of life of men and women on hemodialysis. Baiana Journal of Nursing. 2018;**32**:e24935

[20] Xavier B, Santos I. Patients' feelings and expectations concerning chronic kidney disease and transplant waiting. Journal of Research Care is Fundamental Online. 2012;**4**(4):2832-2840

[21] Orlandini F, Pepino B, Pavarini S, Santos D, Mendiondo M. Assessment of the life expectancy level of elderly people with chronic kidney disease undergoing hemodialysis. Scientific Journal of the School of Nursing at the University of São Paulo. 2012;**46**(4):900-5

[22] Santos ACB, Machado MC, Pereira LR, Abreu JLP, Lyra MB. Association between the level of quality of life and nutritional status in patients undergoing chronic renal hemodialysis. Brazilian Journal of Nephrology. 2013;**35**(4):279-288

[23] Coutinho MPL, Costa FG. Depression and chronic renal failure: A socio-psychological analysis. Psychology & Society. 2015;**27**(2):449-459

[24] Santos I, Rocha R, Berardinelli L. Quality of life of clients on hemodialisys and needs of nursing guidance for self-care. Anna Nery School. 2011;**15**(1): 31-38

[25] Gonçalves CS. Social Representations of Chronic Kidney Disease [master' thesis]. Paraná, Brazil: Postgraduate Program in Nursing, Federal University of Paraná; 2012 p. 82

[26] Ramírez C. Learning to live with a transplanted organ. Scientific Journal of Nursing Science and Care. 2019;**16**(3): 93-102

[27] Pauletto MR, Beuter M, Timm AMB, Santos NO, Roso CC, Jacobi CS. Renal transplant: the perception of patients off waiting list in hemodialyis. Scientific Journal of Nursing at the University of Santa Maria. 2016;**6**(2):154-163

[28] Moreira RA, Borges MS. Profile and level of hope in patients undergoing hemodialysis and peritoneal dialysis. Nursing Cogitare. 2020;**25**:49-59

[29] Araújo A, Almeida E, Lima L, Freitas T, Pinto A. Fall in organ donations and transplants in Ceará in the COVID-19 pandemic: A descriptive study. Journal of Epidemiology and Health Services. April-June 2020, 2021;**30**(1):e2020754

[30] Sartore AC, Grossi SAA. Herth hope index - Instrument adapted and validated to Portuguese. Scientific Journal of the School of Nursing at the University of São Paulo. 2008;**42**(2): 227-232

[31] Reis RP, Lima AP, Lauretino MNB, Bezerra DG. Quality of life and self care of peritoneal dialysis patient compared with hemodialysis: Literature review. Rev eletr. Estácio saúde. 2016;**5**(2):91-106

[32] Cavaco VSJ, José HMG, Louro SPRLP, Ludgero AFA, Martins AFM, Santos MCG. Which is the role of hope in personal health? – Systematic review. Reference Scientific Journal. 2010;**2**(12):93-103

[33] Moreira RA. The feeling of hope in dialysis treatment [master' thesis]. Brasília, Brazil: University of Brasília, Faculty of Health Sciences, Postgraduate Program in Nursing; 2019 p. 115

[34] Roso CC. Self-care for people with chronic kidney failure under conservative treatment [master' thesis]. Rio Grande do Sul, Brazil: Postgraduate Program in Nursing, Federal University of Santa Maria; 2012 p. 120

Section 2

Hemodialysis Routine and Patients Care

Chapter 3

Hemodialysis AV Fistula: What a Radiologist Should Know?

Vaidehi A. Patel

Abstract

Hemodialysis works as a lifeline for end stage renal disease patients. Creation and maintenance of vascular access for dialysis is the mammoth task. Due to increased references related to vascular access; number of complications are faced in pre as well as post operative period of vascular access creation. Ultrasound and color Doppler study play a major role in imaging throughout this period. Pre operative vascular mapping is very crucial to help surgeon to determine the proper site and surgical technique for vascular access creation. Early and delayed post operative complications can also be diagnosed with ultrasound and color Doppler study. Here we have tried to cover all the important points which a radiologist should consider during pre operative vascular mapping and post operative evaluation of vascular access as well as any associated complications.

Keywords: Hemodialysis, Arterio venous fistula, End stage renal disease

1. Introduction

Patients with end stage renal disease (ESDR) on maintenance hemodialysis (MHD) need vascular access to start and continue hemodialysis (HD) as a Renal Replacement Therapy. The Creation and maintenance of vascular access (VA) is a difficult task. With increased references related to VA to radiology department, we face several complications related to preoperative mapping, early postoperative maturity issues along with delayed complications related to VA. We have tried to address issues related to VA formation and maintenance along with providing basic information related to pre and postoperative duplex Ultrasonography (USG). Preoperative Ultrasonography aids to physical examination where patient criteria like obesity, history of access failure, vascular diseases and otherwise difficult examination hinder the clinical assessment of vessels for VA. Development of stenosis or thrombosis leading to failure or immaturity of VA is the main threat in postoperative period. Duplex Ultrasonography allows proper identification of cause of VA failure. Volume flow <500 ml/min or > 50% stenosis correlate with formation of thrombosis within 6 months [1]. Presence of co-morbidity like diabetes and peripheral vascular disease in most of ESRD patients and the always changing local hemodynamic factors complicate the VA commonly. Hence, imaging plays a major role in pre and post operation period for rapid diagnosis and management of VA related complications.

2. Anatomical considerations

VA can be divided in to three types:

Arterio venous fistula (AVF), where anastomosis is surgically formed between artery and vein.

Arterio venous Graft (AVG), where a graft made of poly tetrafluoroethylele (PTFE) is placed between artery and vein.

Central venous catheters (CVC), where a double lumen tube is placed within the central vein usually terminating at or within the right atrium.

The upper extremities are most commonly used for VA. AVF or AVG is made by connecting a vein with artery or interposition of synthetic graft between them which provides a high flow circuit for percutaneous cannulation for hemodialysis. A mature AVF is better than AVG in given higher patency rates, lesser infection chances and reduced maintainace. Generally, the upper limb is used to create such communication. The Non dominant upper limb is the first choice to facilitate daily activities with

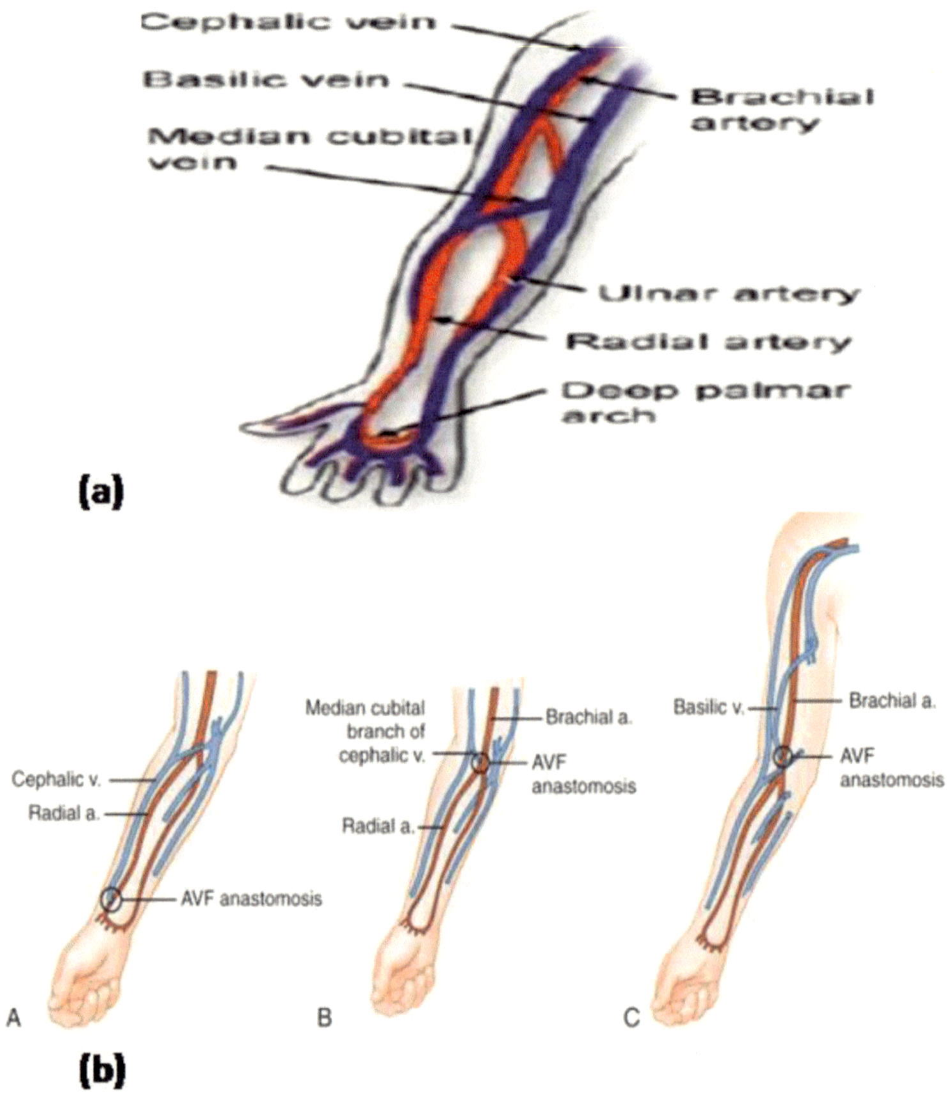

Figure 1.
Upper limb vascular anatomy (a) and (b) various types of AVF [3, 4].

dominant limb while providing adequate time to VA for maturation. Usually, AVF is considered in forearm to preserve the proximal vessels for future if required. Likewise, AVG is preferred in non dominant arm rather than forearm. AVF can be created through a surgical anastomosis between vessels where both the vessels may be in their normal position or the distal end of vein may be transpositioned more superficially to facilitate cannulation, while in Translocation, the entire vein is moved and anastomosis is done.

So, the preferred type and sites of anastomosis would be - forearm AVF > arm AVF > arm AVG > thigh AVG in respect to available vessels.

The most preferred type of AVF which is *Radio-cephalic fistula* made in forearm near wrist can also fail to mature in elder patients with underlying vascular or diabetic etiology [2]. *Brachio cephalic AVF* is usually made in antecubital fossa providing benefits of ease of cannulation due to larger surface area (**Figure 1**) [3, 4]. However it poses a major complication – steal syndrome (*will be discussed later*). As basilic vein is less commonly accessed for venipuncture, it is usually better preserved and is less commonly involved in post venipuncture phlebitis in comparison to cephalic vein. However, Brachio-basilic AVF in arm involves dual surgical procedure, difficult to cannulate due to medial location of basilic vein and more prone to infections.

Central venous catheters (CVC) provide short term access in emergency conditions, but they are associated with higher rates of failure, infection and mortality. Patients switching to AVF or AVG from CVCs have almost 50% reduction in mortality [5]. Moreover, previous CVC placement poses a risk of central venous stenosis due to endothelial injury and thrombosis caused by them.

3. Role of radiology

According to Dialysis Outcome Quality Initiative (DOQI) guidelines, AVF is preferred over AVG due to its greater lifespan and reduced incidence of infection. Detailed imaging of vascular anatomy prior to AVF creation provides good evaluation of veins that may be suitable for the creation of AVF, particularly in patients with previous failed AVF and/or history of CVC placement. Detailed preoperative imaging helps the surgeon to choose suitable efferent vein and surgical technique (in the form of AVF or AVG and transposition or translocation in AVF). Also, it helps to select the most functional vein which helps in decreasing postoperative failure and complications (**Figure 2**). However, a considerable number of AVFs fail to mature and in those patients, Ultrasonography can evaluate the etiology of immaturity. If the exact etiology is known, the role of Intervention (angioplasty of a stenosis) or Surgery (AVF revision or accessory vein ligation) can be cleared. VAs are commonly imaged by Ultrasonography and color doppler study (CDI); however other modalities like DSA, MRI and CT scan can also be used as and when necessary. But, we will focus on various aspects related to Ultrasonography and color doppler study in pre and postoperative imaging of VAs. Catheters in situ, overlying dressing, open wounds, Severe Edema and hematoma can hinder the visibility in USG.

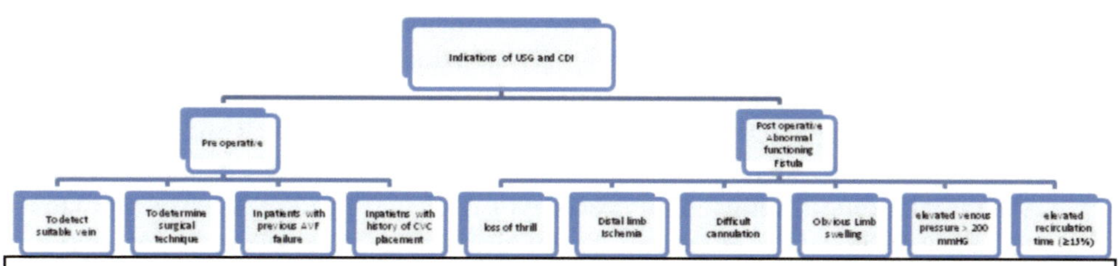

Flow chart shows preoperative and Postoperative indications for USG and CD Imaging.

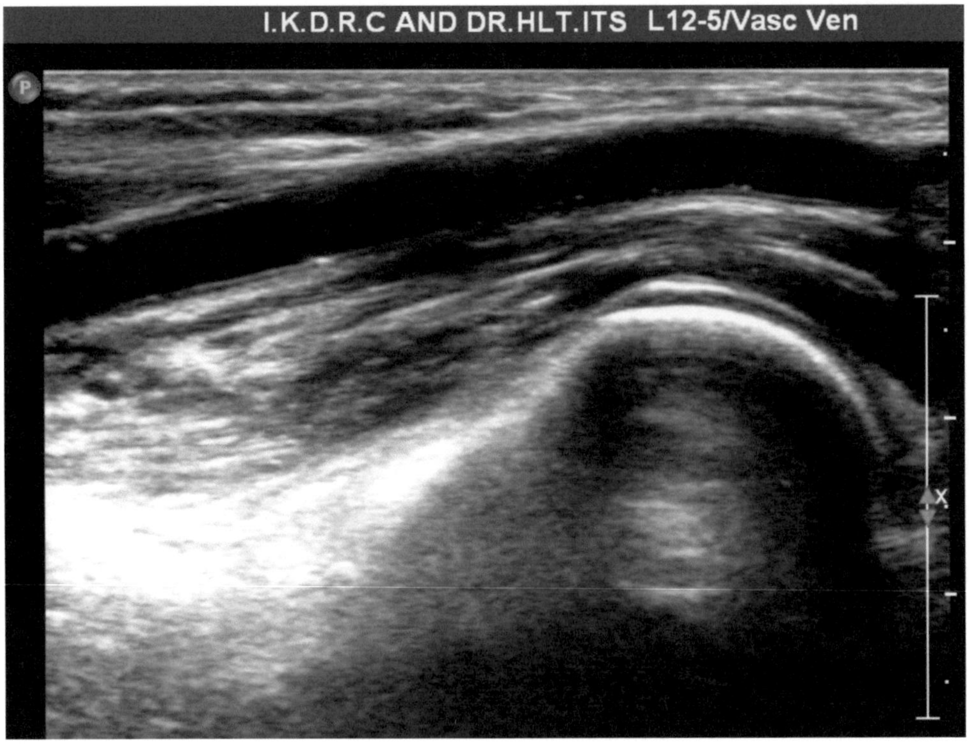

Figure 2.
Gray mode USG image showing minimal intimal wall thickening and multiple tiny flecks of calcification within the wall of brachial artery.

3.1 Preoperative evaluation of AVF/AVG

High resolution linear transducer (≥ 9 MHz) is used for vascular mapping. For ease of description, vessels towards shoulder will be considered proximal and towards the wrist will be considered distal vessels. The scanning is done at room temperature to avoid vasoconstriction in cooler temperature. Warm blankets or warm compression can be used if necessary. The patient should be relaxed and rested in sitting or supine position whichever is comfortable with proximal tourniquet binding. The non dominant arm is assessed first and is placed in extended position along his sides or on any support (like pillow) according to patient's position. The upper limb should be abducted and externally rotated for better visualization.

B mode axial plane imaging is ideal for evaluating vascular anatomy and to evaluate their diameter as well as wall thickness. Arteries are evaluated for presence of any intimo-medial thickening, wall calcification or stenosis. Presence of calcification in arterial wall hinders its distensibility and may contribute towards dysfunction (**Figure 3**). Veins are evaluated for compressibility (denoting to patency) and the depth of anterior venous wall from the level of skin. Color doppler study of arteries evaluates color filling of lumen and excludes luminal narrowing or thrombosis. Spectral waveform excludes any distal occlusion or vascular disease. Color doppler study of veins evaluates venous phasicity and respiratory variations.

Usually the imaging is started from Radial artery. The vessel wall and internal diameter of radial artery at forearm are assessed. If the diameter is not at least 2 mm at wrist, the radial artery is not used for creation of AVF. If the radial artery is satisfactory, cephalic vein at wrist is evaluated. Brachial artery is also evaluated for possible

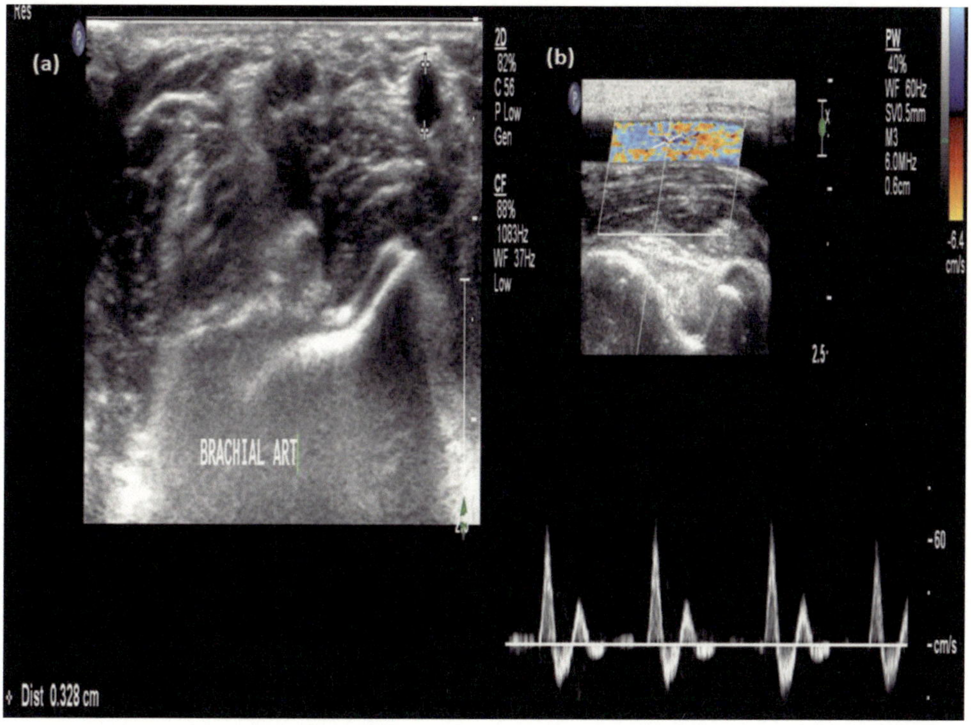

Figure 3.
(a) Gray mode image showing brachial artery at elbow with internal lumen diameter 3.2 mm, (b) CDI study showing normal color flow with triphasic waveform.

arm fistula placement. All the peripheral arteries show Triphasic waveform on CDI study (**Figure 4**). For evaluation of cephalic vein at wrist, tourniquet is tightened in proximal forearm and the distal limb is percussed for about 3 minutes. The main idea behind tourniquet and percussion is that the veins capable of distending up to 2.5 mm will be preferred for AVF due to their distensibility during higher venous pressures. Veins with diameter smaller than 2 mm will not distend up to adequate diameter in most cases. Cephalic vein is then assessed for continuity up to proximal forearm and if its adequate, then the tourniquet is shifted to a more proximal level. If the cephalic vein is narrow in caliber, discontinuous, stenotic or shows thrombus or thick wall, it is not adequate for AVF creation. Branch points must be thoroughly imaged, as they may show narrowing below 2.5 mm in veins. After the forearm is assessed, the vein should be traced up to axilla to evaluate the sites of deep venous communication. Evaluation of neck veins should also a routine practice in upper limb mapping as any abnormality in neck veins can contribute to future AVF failure. If cephalic vein is not adequate for AVF, basilic vein is assessed in the same manner (**Figures 5** and **6**).

If forearm vessels are not promising for wrist AVF creation, AVF at elbow is considered and brachial artery is imaged. Brachial artery internal diameter is measured above its bifurcation in to radial and ulnar arteries, which must be ≥2 mm. The cephalic vein is then assessed at antecubital fossa. Cephalic vein must be at least 2.5 mm in diameter and must extend about 2 cm distal to antecubital fossa. If cephalic vein is not suitable, basilic vein is considered and it must extend to about 4 cm proximal to antecubital fossa for AVF formation. Chronically thrombosed cephalic vein is a very frequent finding in ESRD patients due to frequent venipuncture. Cephalic vein appears narrow with thick walls and appears cord like with no internal color flow in such cases (**Figure 7**). However, sometimes median cubital vein may also be used as

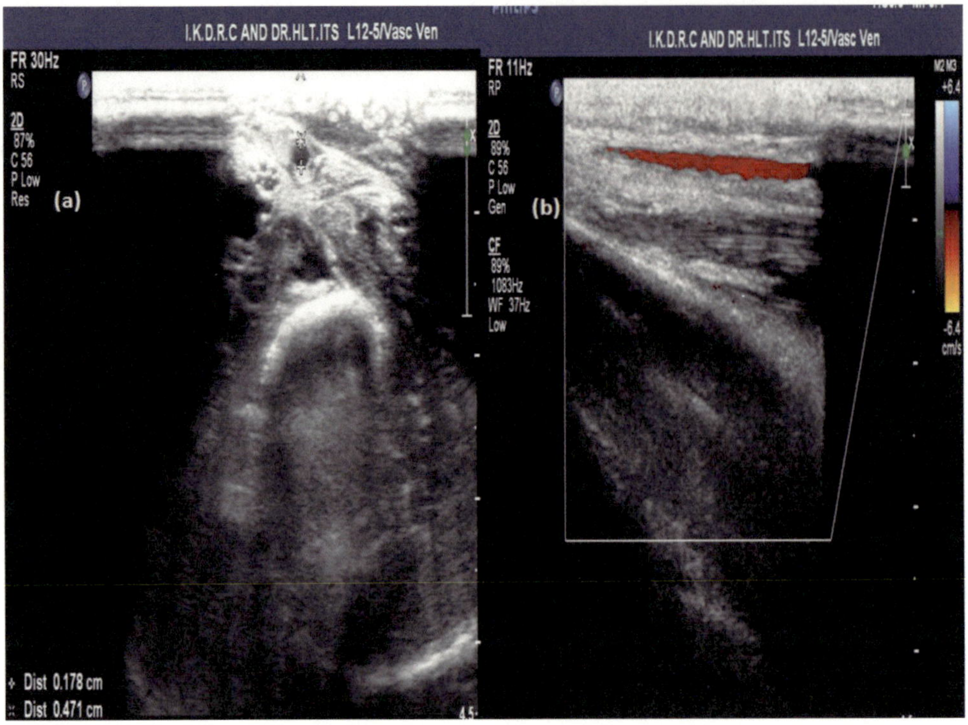

Figure 4.
(a) Gray mode image showing narrow Cephalic vein in forearm with internal lumen diameter 1.8 mm and depth from skin level measuring about 4.7 mm and (b) patent lumen on color doppler study.

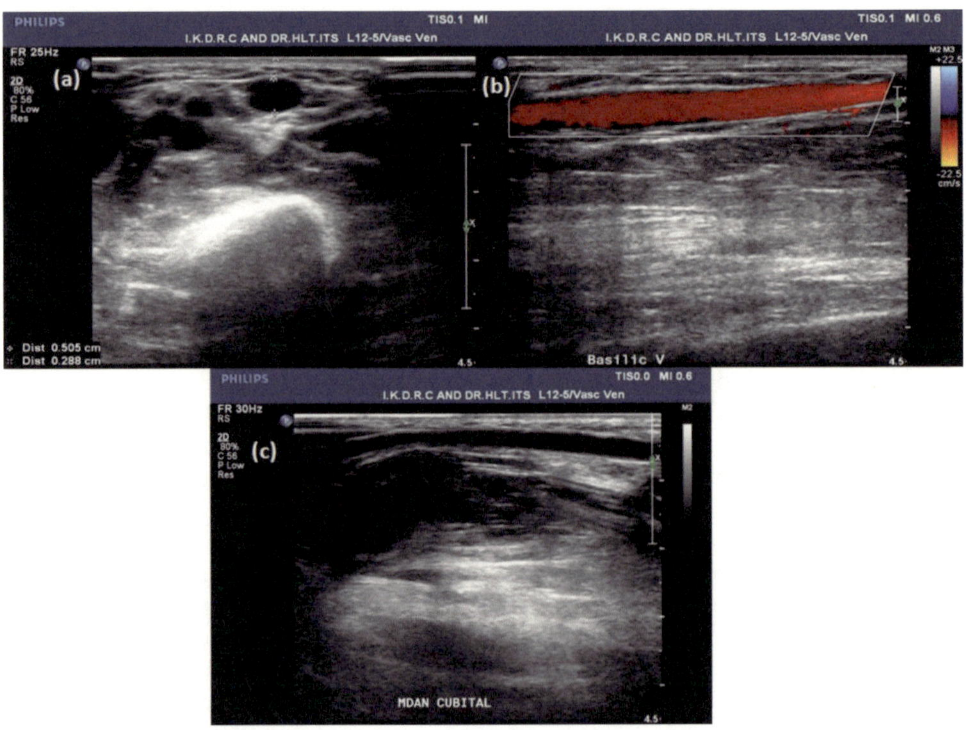

Figure 5.
(a) Gray mode image showing basilic vein at elbow with internal lumen diameter 2.8 mm and depth from skin level measuring about 5.0 mm, (b) CDI study showing normal color flow, (c) gray scale image showing normal median cubital vein in cubital fossa.

DOI: http://dx.doi.org/10.5772/intechopen.100485

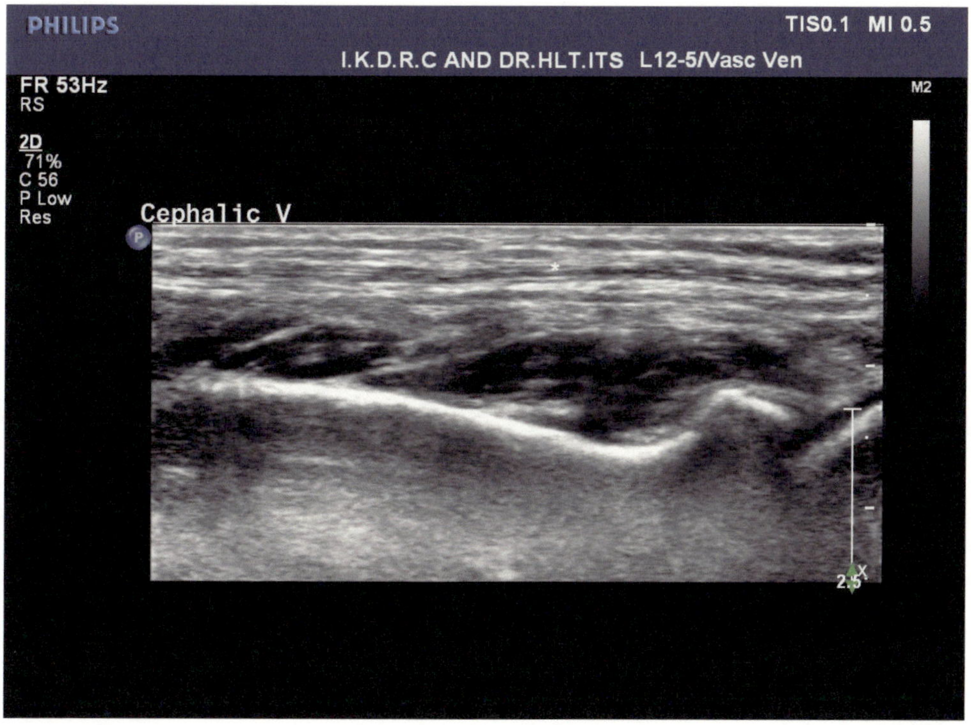

Figure 6.
Gray mode image showing chronically thrombosed narrow cord like Cephalic vein (*).

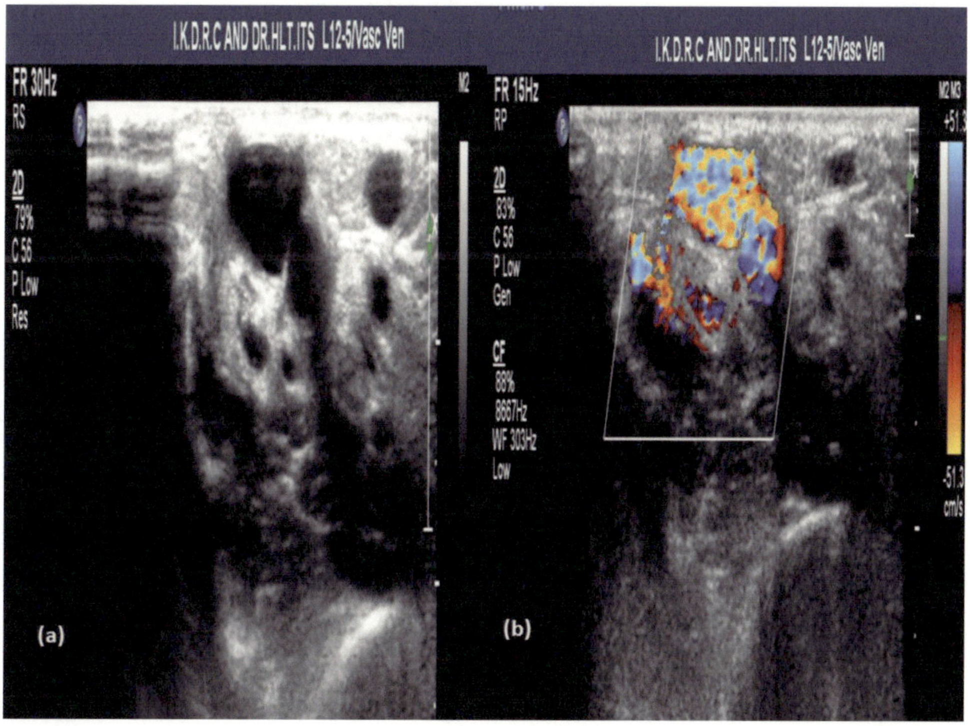

Figure 7.
(a) Gray mode image showing AVF (b) CDI study showing normal aliasing color flow within the AVF.

an alternative as it courses close to brachial artery. In any case, considerable length of patent vein is needed for the surgical procedure as well as during dialysis.

3.1.1 Important points for preoperative evaluation

- Prefer Non- dominant limb (if possible, preserve non dominant arm from the first consultation only)
- Consider the site of AVF placement as per recommendation and evaluate accordingly
- Arteries- evaluate anatomy, branching pattern, continuity, wall thickness, presence of calcification, internal diameter
- Veins- evaluate anatomy, lumen patency, wall thickening, internal diameter, depth from the skin surface, any focal areas of stenosis, branching points and regions of drainage in to deep veins. Neck veins are also evaluated for any possible thrombosis or stenosis
- If the cephalic vein in arm is not suitable for AVF, still cephalic vein in forearm can be used for AVF provided it drains in to brachial or basilic vein through adequate median cubital or other branch.
- Areas of focal stenosis should be looked for at any accessory vein branches which may significantly affect blood flow in AVF later.
- Normal diameter sized cephalic vein with deeper location (depth > 5 mm) may be difficult for palpation later for needle insertion. So the surgeon and patient must clear about future requirement of superficialization.
- High radial artery branching from brachial or axillary artery is a common variant that must be sought for because if present, it may contribute towards increased arterial steal.

3.2 Postoperative evaluation of AVF

According to National Kidney Foundation's Kidney Disease Outcomes Quality Initiative (KDOQI), clinical examination remains the key to determination of maturation. However, USG and CDI prove reliable for surveillance assessment and to find causes of immaturation and complications if any. USG evaluation of AVF is done with high resolution (≥9 mHz) probe without tourniquet. Minimal pressure is applied while scanning with generous amount of ultrasound gel for proper visualization.

The evaluation of AVF starts with clinical examination, where the AVF is palpated for a possible thrill which denotes its proper working. Scanning is then initiated from the feeding artery in axial and Saggital views. The artery is traced towards the draining vein and overall anatomy is evaluated. Feeding artery adjacent to AVF is examined for any wall thickening, lumen patency and areas of stenosis in B mode scanning. Color doppler study is used to see uniform color filling and aliasing color flow like AVF (**Figure 8**). Pulse wave doppler is used for noting biphasic waveform in artery instead of usual Triphasic waveform seen in preoperative artery (**Figure 9**). Peak systolic velocity (PSV) in the feeding artery increases to about 9 to 10 fold in comparison to pre AVF state in mature AVF. PSV is measured in the artery at the level of AVF and 2 cm proximal to it.

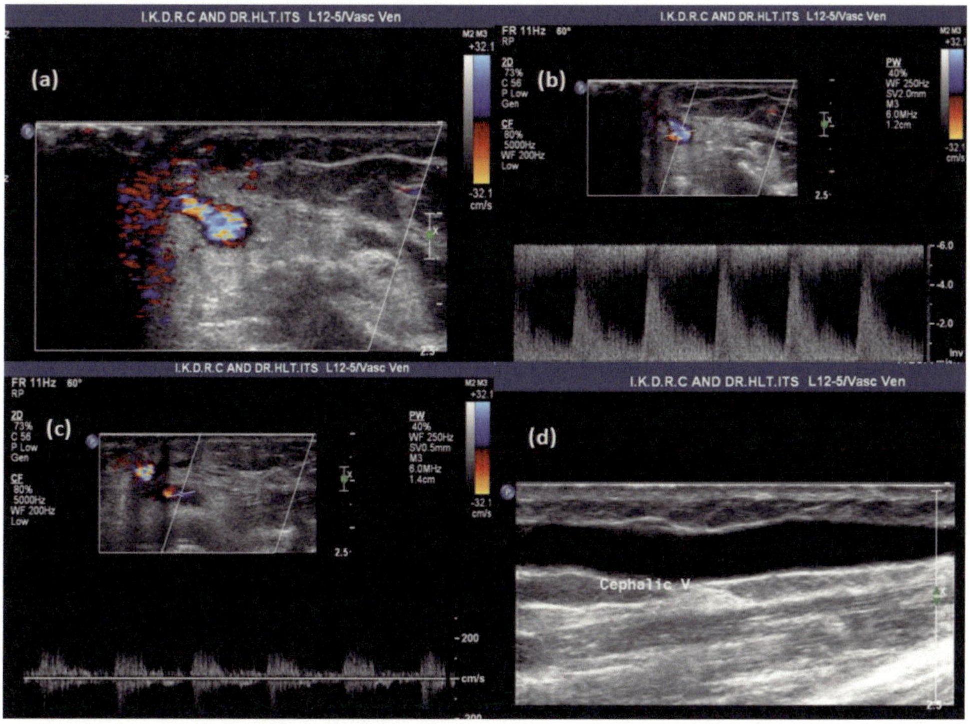

Figure 8.
(a) CDI image showing working AVF with colorailising, (b) CDI study showing normal spectral waveform with high PSV within the AVF, (c) normal post AVF biphasic waveform in brachial artery, (d) mild dilated cephalic vein with patent lumen.

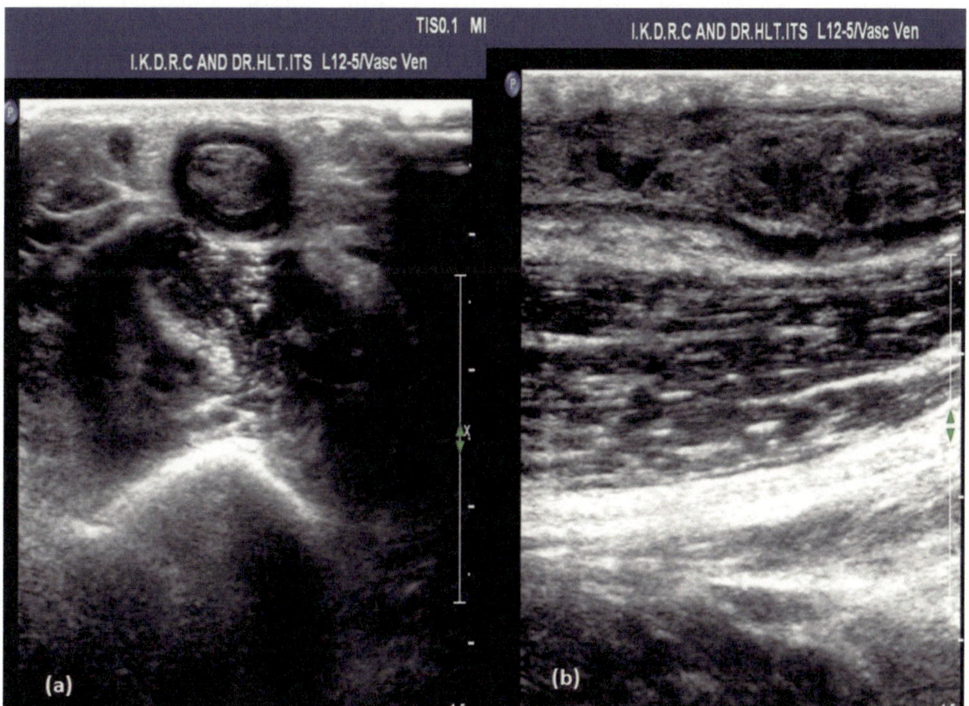

Figure 9.
Gray scale image showing complete thrombus in cephalic vein in (a) axial and (b) longitudinal scans.

3.2.1 PSV ratio: PSV at the anastomosis / PSV 2 cm proximal/distal to AVF

PSV ratio is useful to exclude stenosis. Blood flow is measured within the AVF in mid part. Measuring blood flow volume warrants specific technique where it must be measured in continuous nontapering segment of draining vein about 10 cm from anastomosis. It is measured in middle of the lumen with maximum gate and not more than 60 degree insonation angle. Time averaged mean velocity should be counted for 3 cardiac cycles and then internal diameter of the vessel is measured. According to these parameters, scanner calculates the volume flow in ml per minutes.

3.2.2 Volume flow: time averaged velocity X vessel cross sectional area

AVF itself shows aliasing color flow within it. Blood flow more than 500 to 600 mL/min is required in mature AVF along with the maximum venous diameter about 5 to 6 mm. Presence of both of these criteria confirms maturity in about 95% of AVF. National Kidney Foundation's Kidney Disease Outcomes Quality Initiative clinical practice guidelines defines a "rule of sixes," for maturation of AVF stating that it should have blood flow of ≥600 ml/min, a diameter of ≥6 mm, and a depth of ≤6 mm from the surface of the skin. Along with scanning of AVF, feeding artery and draining veins; evaluation of deep and neck veins should also be a routine practice in Postoperative imaging to rule out any complication at early stage.

3.2.3 Important points for postoperative evaluation of AVF

- Imaging of AVF in Postoperative 1st or 2nd day is counted as 1st scan followed by 2nd week and 6th week scanning
- Tourniquet is not used with minimal pressure and generous amount of gel
- Maximum gate with not more than 60 degree insonation angle used in the middle of vessel
- Feeding artery, AVF itself and draining veins are evaluated and they show aliasing color flow. Puncture sites are also evaluated for possible thrombosis.
- Vessels looked for patency and regions of narrowing
- Blood flow measured in mid part of AVF and continuous non tapering segment of draining vein about 10 cm from anastomosis
- Blood flow of ≥600 ml/min, a diameter of ≥6 mm, and a depth of ≤6 mm from the surface of the skin are ideal for mature AVF.
- Deep veins of upper limb should also be seen to rule out early deep vein thrombosis
- Neck veins are also evaluated for possible steal syndrome, obstruction or thrombosis
- Large vein branches are also looked for within first 10 cm of draining veins, which eventually decrease the blood flow in AVF contributing to immaturity.

Due to higher incidence of infection, stenosis and pseudoaneurysm; AVGs are less preferred over AVF. Preoperative vascular mapping for AVF is done in the same manner as in AVF. AVGs are assessed by USG or CDI if palpable focal mass is seen adjacent to AVG. In such cases there may be graft stenosis. CDI differentiates hematoma from pseudoaneurysm. Symptomatic AVGs should be referred for angiography where it may be treated with angioplasty with or without stent placement if stenosis is present. However, in some cases graft degeneration also causes focal area of larger diameter presenting as palpable mass. In Postoperative evaluation of AVG, feeding artery, AVG, arterial and venous anastomosis and draining vein are evaluated. In loop grafts, identification of direction of blood flow is first step to facilitate identification of arterial and venous limb. The PSV is calculated at 2 cm proximal to arterial anastomosis (seen in the feeding artery) and 2 cm distal to venous anastomosis (seen in the AVG). If visible stenosis is present, PSV ratio (described earlier) is calculated at anastomosis. In presence of upper arm AVG, subclavian vein may show monophasic waveform even if there is no central stenosis. If the venous outflow from the graft is greater than the feeding arterial capacity, arterial steal occurs distal to arterial anastomosis [5].

4. Complications

Rate of complications is much lesser in AVF as compared to AVG or CVC. However they do occur in 1/3rd cases [2] and are addressed here. Most commonly seen complications of AVF are thrombosis, aneurysm, infection, stenosis, steal syndrome and heart failure. Complications are divided in early and late. However, fistula failure also occurs and that may be classified as primary (fistula that fails to mature even before cannulation) and secondary (delayed failure or after any intervention).

4.1 Early complications/early failure

It is defined as AVF which fails to mature or unable for use up to 3 months after creation. Causes of early failure may be related to inadequate arterialinflow, stenosis at anastomosis or outflow issues due to underlying fibrosis of vein. Various causes for early failure or complications are listed below:

- Demographic factors: Age, obesity, female, history of diabetes or peripheral vascular
- Disease
- Size of draining vein along with reduced distensibility
- Development of collateral circulation

4.2 Late complications/late failure

Fistula Failure occurring after 3 months duration after creation of AVF are classified as late failure. Various complications are seen like; Stenosis, aneurysm, steal syndrome, infection, cardiac failure, venous hypertension, median nerve injury.

4.2.1 Thrombosis

Thrombosis is noted within the fistula in early as well as late Postoperative period. Early thrombosis is most often related to an inflow issues and late thrombosis due to an outflow stenosis. Either of these can result in thrombosis of the fistula if left untreated. Difficult cannulation, sudden reduction in VA flow or a new onset low flow in VA should trigger the possible diagnosis of thrombosis. Physical examination may show absent thrill in AVF and pulsatile anastomosis is felt. On USG and CDI, the affected vein may be dilated and show echogenic thrombus filling the lumen with no internal color filling. Partial thrombus is also seen. Needle insertion sites should be evaluated carefully as there may be partial thrombus at these sites. In case of thrombosis in draining vein, AVF itself shows no evidence of aliasing color flow and the feeding artery shows triphasic normal spectral waveform instead of biphasic spectral waveform seen in working AVF.

4.2.2 Stenosis

It is often due to outflow stenosis. Venous stenosis is more commonly seen in AVF than AVG. However, it is common cause of failure. Swelling of upper limb, prolonged bleeding after dialysis, difficult cannulation and/or slow flow are common symptoms of venous stenosis. In radio cephalic AVF, inflow lesions due to inadequate arterial flow is confirmed by negative arterial pressure during HD session and physical examination by pulse augmentation. In brachio cephalic AVF, cephalic arch stenosis is very commonly (in up to 77% cases) seen causing failure. Cephalic arch is the final bend in cephalic vein when it enters in to axillary vein. Cephalic arch stenosis causes swelling in head and neck, high venous pressure with thrombosis. Venous or arterial stenosis can be successfully managed by angioplasty [2]. Cephalic arch stenosis warrants stent placement due to its elasticity and resistant nature to repeated angioplasty. During pre and Postoperative scanning, entire length of vessels should be traced for any possible stenosis or narrowing. PSV ratio is measured in feeding artery at the level of AVF and 2 cm proximal to it.

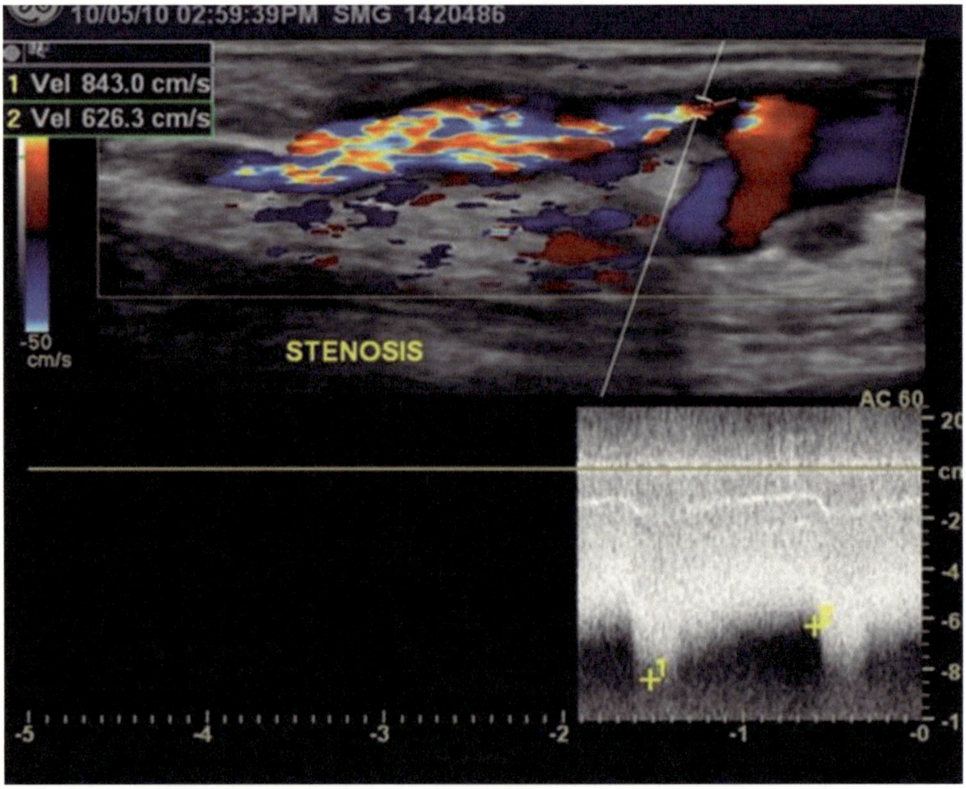

Figure 10.
Gray scale image showing stenosis with post stenotic turbulent color flow and marked elevated PSV and EDV [6].

If the PSV ratio is ≥3.0 and PSV is >400 cm/sec, stenosis is present. If the draining vein is visibly narrow, PSV is measured at stenosis and at 2 cm caudal to stenosis. If the PSV ratio is ≥2.0, stenosis is considered (**Figure 10**). Most frequent site of AVF stenosis is adjacent to anastomosis. Presence of adequate collaterals, low systemic pressure, poor Dopplerinsonation angle and central venous stenosis are some of the factors which can hinder the diagnosis of stenosis. However the degree of stenosis is not absolute in AVF failure prediction.

4.2.3 Aneurysm

Repeated cannulation at repetitive sites or turbulent blood flow due to stenosis is the major causes of formation of aneurysm. It is seen in about 5 to 7% cases. Physiological and esthetic complications due to aneurysm lead to surgery in many cases and may cause failure subsequently. Increased infection risk and prolonged bleeding after dialysis along with complex surgery are common associated complications of aneurysm. On scanning, outpouching with or without color flow is seen arising from vessels (**Figure 11**). Most common site is the needle insertion site. The aneurysm may show to and frocolor flow and peripheral thrombosis. In case of thrombosis, patent lumen commonly shows color flow. The entire length of vessel should be traced as finding more than one aneurysms is not uncommon. Totally thrombosed aneurysm sometime look like old hematoma and in such cases proper history and careful evaluation in terms of connection with the vessel wall should be done. Internal color flow can clear the doubts in such cases. Treatment of aneurysm consists of its prevention in the form of careful cannulation techniques and surgical correction techniques [2].

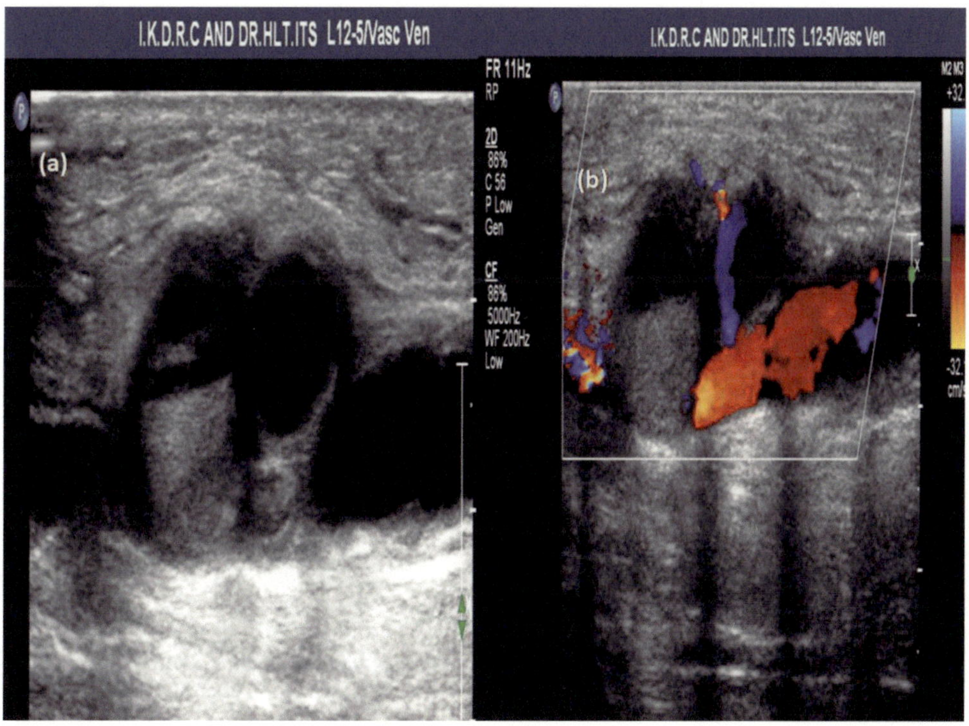

Figure 11.
(a) Gray scale image showing aneurysm arising from brachial artery in mid arm with peripheral thrombosis and (b) CDI study showing color flow in patent lumen.

4.2.4 Infection

Infection affects AVF (20% of all complications in AVF) less commonly than AVG (10 fold increased risk of infection in comparison to AVF). Perivascular cellulitis manifesting as localized redness and oedema is seen in cases of infection of AVF. Physical examination readily detects presence of infection. So, USG or CDI is not very commonly advised but it the sign symptoms persist after antibiotic regime, imaging can be advised. In Gray mode USG, subcutaneous oedema with or without fluid collections at AVF site is noted. The AVF is working in most of the cases. In cases of associated thrombosis, AVF may be non working with presence of thrombosis in draining vein or AVF. If associated aneurysm, hematoma or abscess are present, meticulous imaging and prompt treatment in form of surgical excision or drainage is done [6].

4.2.5 Steal syndrome

Distal hypo-perfusion of the limb in case of severe peripheral vascular disease due to pulling of arterial blood flow in AVF causes steal syndrome. Failure of adequate collateral formation and/or excessive blood flow is the main causes of symptomatic steal. About 3 to 8% cases may present with steal syndrome [7]. Brachiocephalic AVF tend to cause steal more than radio-cephalic AVF. Hand ischemia, pain, numbness are some of the symptoms where steal syndrome may be present. AVF shows normal color flow and high PSV.

For arterial steal, radial artery at wrist is usually examined. In complete arterial steal, direction of flow distal to the graft is reversed, however in partial steal, the spectral waveform becomes biphasic. Steal syndrome is confirmed if gentle compression of graft reverses the direction of flow and normal spectral waveform is achieved (**Figure 12**). Symptomatic steal may require graft ligation. However, asymptomatic steal is also seen which warrants no clinical significance.

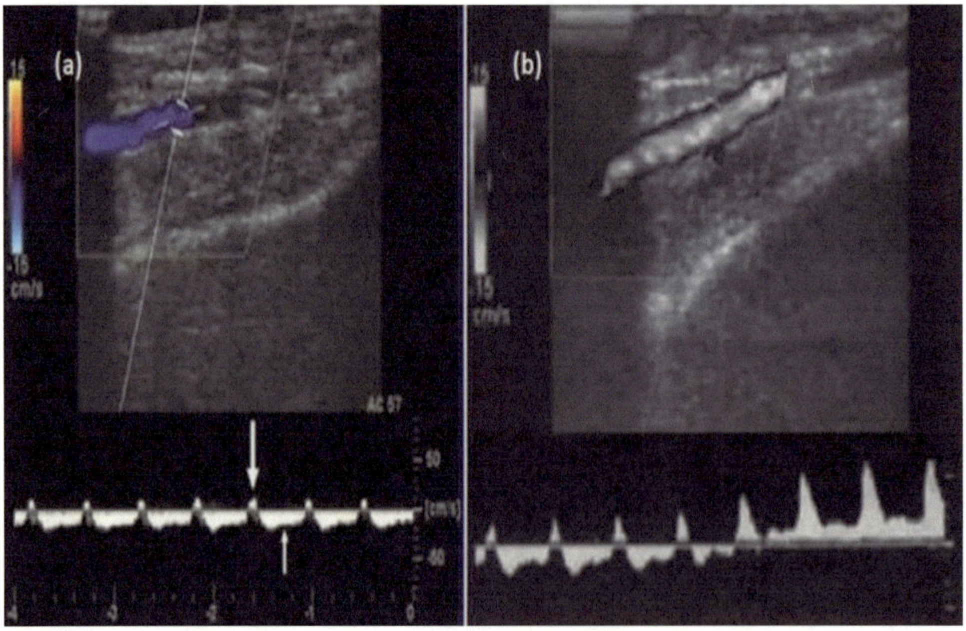

Figure 12.
(a) CDI image showing antegrade flow during systole and retrograde flow during diastole in radial artery distal to anastomosis (b) on gentle compression of AVF, elevated systolic flow and diastolic flow is noted confirming arterial steal syndrome [8].

Other complications like cardiac failure, venous hypertension and median nerve injury are also noted in relation to AVF. However, they are not very common and role of radiology is not prevalent. Venous hypertension may be seen as reversal of blood flow in color doppler study. Median nerve injury may occur from ischemic injury due to steal syndrome or direct compression of median nerve due to hematoma or amyloid deposition in late phases of AVF. In such cases, radiology can evaluate the primary etiology.

5. Conclusion

This chapter has reviewed important aspects of pre and Postoperative evaluation of hemodialysis AVF. USG and CDI are principal imaging modality due to various advantages like easy availability, non invasive, non-ionizing and cheap modality. A detailed protocol for performing and interpreting USG and CDI studies for VA has been developed through our vast experience and we have tried to provide a proper performa for VA evaluation.

Acknowledgements

I want to pay heartfelt gratitudeto my patients and fellow clinicians for providing us a wide experience in this field. I also want to thank Ms Jyotsana Suthar, our librarian for the technical help throughout the time during the process of writing this chapter.

Author details

Vaidehi A. Patel
Department of Radio Diagnosis, Institute of Kidney Diseases and Research Centre and Dr. H.L. Trivedi Institute of Transplantation Sciences, Gujarat University of Transplantation Sciences, Asarwa, Ahmedabad, Gujarat, India

*Address all correspondence to: drvaidehipandya@gmail.com

References

[1] B.S.Strauch, R.S. O'Connell, K.L. Geoly et al. Forecasting thrombosis of vascular access with Doppler color flow imaging. American Journal of Kidney Diseases 1992, vol 19, no. 6, pp. 554-557.

[2] Technical Problems in Patients on Hemodialysis, edited by Maria Goretti Penido. "Hemodialysis Access: The Fistula" by Mary Hammes. Published by InTech, JanezaTrdline 9, 51000 Rijeka, Croatia. Page 17-34.

[3] Deklunder G, Dauzat M, Boivin V, Sédiri I. *Exploration des vaisseaux du membre supérieur: Doppler et échotomographie*. EMC-Radiologie 2004; 1(6): 632-646

[4] Introduction to vascular Ultrasonography; 6th Edition edited by John S. Pellerito and Joseph F. Polak. Ultrasound evaluation before and after hemodialysis access by Michelle L Robbin, Mark E Lockhart. Published by Elsevier, Philadelphia, PA. Page no 281-293

[5] Eion A Murphy, Rose A. Ross, Robert G. Jones et al. Imaging in Vascular access. Cardiovascular Engineering and Technology. Vol 8, No. 3, September 2017 pp. 255-272.

[6] Victoria Teodorescu, Susan Gustavson, Harry Schanzer. Duplex Ultrasound Evaluation of Hemodialysis Access: A Detailed Protocol. Int J Nephro. 2012;2012:508956. PMID: 22848824

[7] Most Important Chronic Complications of Arteriovenous Fistulas for Hemodialysis Radojica Stolic Med Princ Pract. 2013;22:220-228

[8] Cengiz Yilmaz, Kaan Ozcan, Nazif Erkan. Dialysis access-associated steal syndrome presenting as bidirectional flow at duplex Doppler ultrasound. Am J Roentgenol. 2009 Dec;193(6):W568. PMID: 19933633

Chapter 4

Exhaustion of Vascular Accesses for Haemodialysis: Access by Thrombosed Vein

Arturo Rafael Vizcarra

Abstract

I will describe, especially to professionals involved in vascular access, how recently occluded veins can be recanalized to implant a haemodialysis catheter. We recommend that it be a permanent one.

Keywords: exhaustion, vascular accesses, haemodialysis, access, thrombosed vein

1. Introduction

The depletion of vascular accesses for haemodialysis is seen in some patients who reach this situation due to multiple causes [1, 2] such as procoagulant factors, lack of good management of their accesses, lack of resources, etc.

In these cases, the skills of the surgical team to respond must be technically sharpened.

When a patient is without vascular access and cannot dialyze, it is an extreme situation.

It is understood that a patient does not have vascular access when not even a catheter can be implanted to be able to dialyze.

That is, there is occlusion or inability to progress a catheter through the following veins:

1. Internal jugulars

2. External jugulars

3. Subclavian

4. Femoral

1.1 Options for implanting a catheter in these conditions

Where do wrong decisions bring bad results? The following options are the most common ones for implanting a permanent catheter. In some cases, this catheter can be connected to a prosthesis to make a fistula.

There are not many options to do this; some of the possible options are listed below:

a. Translumbarpuncture of the inferior vena cava [3, 4]

b. Direct puncture of the superior vena cava [5]

c. Transliver puncture [6],

d. Sternotomy or thoracotomy for direct access to the right atrium.

All of these options are not the subject of this chapter.

2. Implant a catheter through a thrombosed vein

I recommend that these practices be done by a surgeon who often performs haemodialysis accesses, or by an operator in conjunction with a surgeon, so that if a complication occurs he/she can resolve it or use a different tactic.

There must be an operating room equipped with an echo doppler equipment, good quality fluoroscopy, specialised human resources, a variety of guide wires, catheters, dilators, and a complete set of cardiovascular surgery [7] (**Figure 1**).

Given this situation and the fact that the patient is young, I implant catheters through any of the veins mentioned above, either because they have a central occlusion or because they are directly thrombosed throughout their entire course. Often I have been able to implant catheters in those with recent occlusion (**Figures 2–4**).

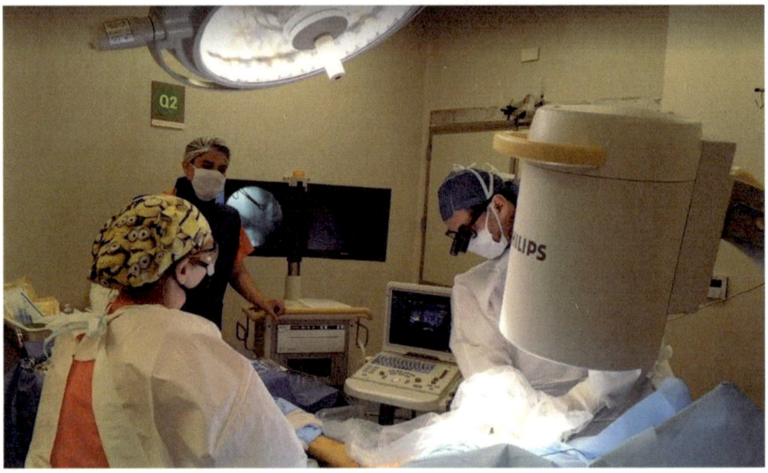

Figure 1.
Operating room, equipped with doppler echo, fluoroscopy, surgical fields, surgeon's assistants, complete surgical instruments.

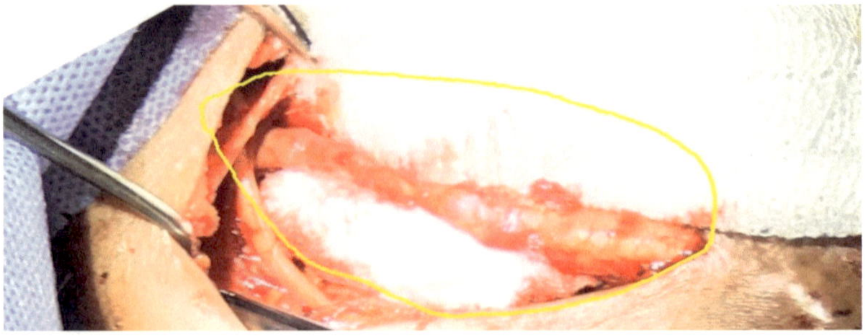

Figure 2.
Occluded vein, with long stenosis, dissected for the repair of an arteriovenous fistula for haemodialysis.

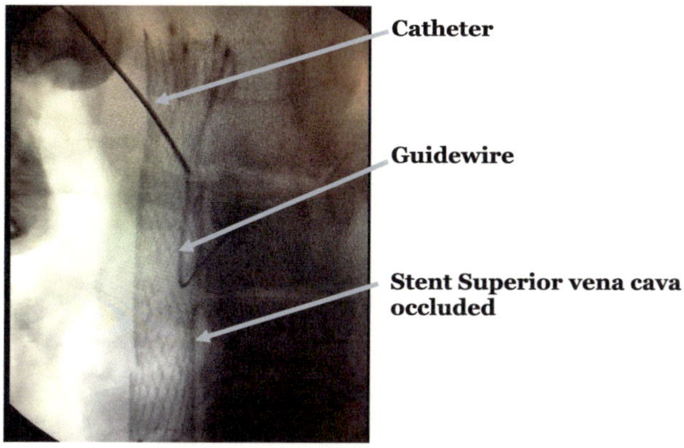

Figure 3.
Old occlusion of the superior vena cava with a stent also occluded, a guidewire, catheter and stent can be seen; it was not possible to pass; in this case, the femoral vein with recent occlusion is accessed.

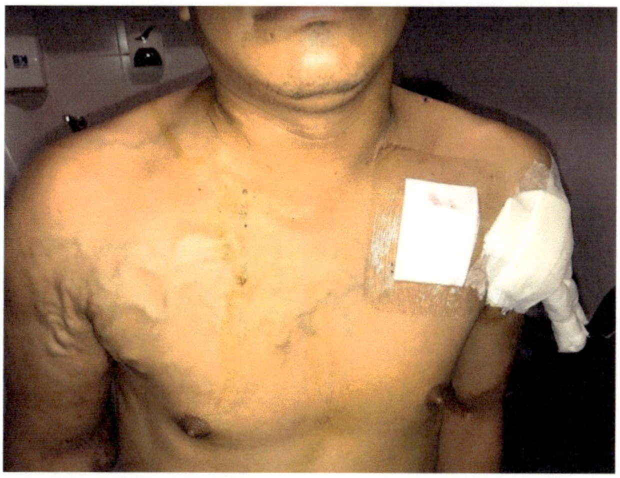

Figure 4.
This case of recent occlusion of the innominate vein and left subclavian could be passed. The right side shows abundant collateral venous circulation for a long-time occlusion.

Occluded veins with a long time of evolution is usually fibrosed and it is difficult or impossible to cross with the guide wire.

2.1 I'm going to talk to you about this topic very specifically

These patients, usually in the superior veins, have had a stent placed, **Figure 3**, or an angioplasty done previously, which makes it even more difficult.

Less frequent in the lower limbs, which is reserved as a last option.

2.2 So what is the basis of puncturing thrombosed veins to be able to pass with a catheter?

The rationale is that veins, especially those recently occluded and therefore thrombosed, at some point have loose tissues, enough to pass with a wire guide, which can be helped with catheters or dilators.

The recent occlusion of the vein in arteriovenous fistulas in repair surgeries is shown. Through the small hole or loose tissue, seen in the images, the passage can be opened to advance a guide wire and then a catheter when a thrombosed vein is punctured (**Figures 5–8**).

All manoeuvres must be done carefully.

In order to move forward, you have to take the time that is necessary.

It is recommended that surgeons do this procedure, because if there is any complication at the moment that requires surgery, it can be solved by the operator himself.

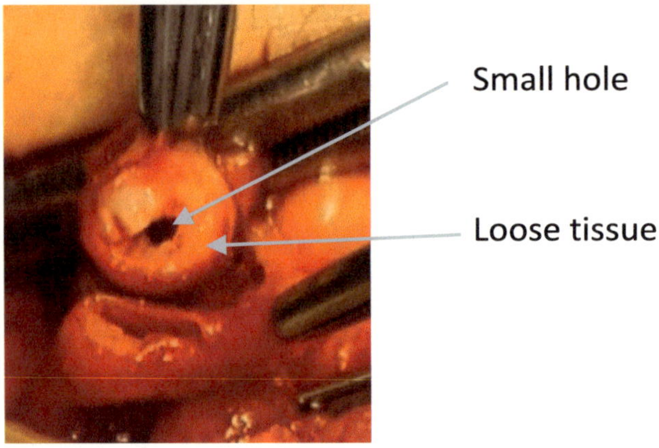

Figure 5.
Recently occluded basilica vein; in AVF repair; you can see that there is a small hole.

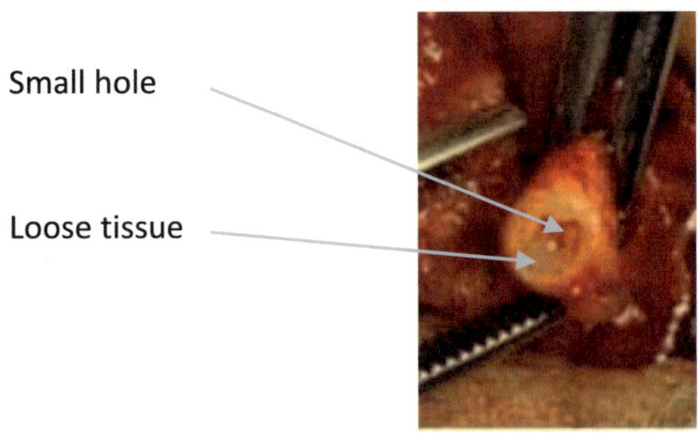

Figure 6.
Recently occluded femoral vein; in AVF repair; you can see that there is a small hole.

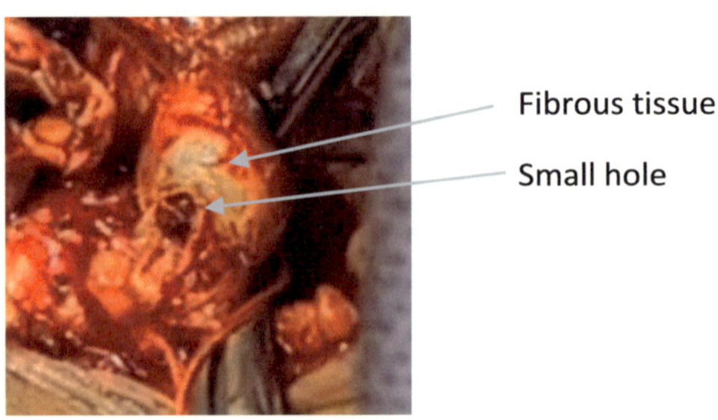

Figure 7.
Recently occluded axillary vein; in AVF repair; you can see that there is a small hole.

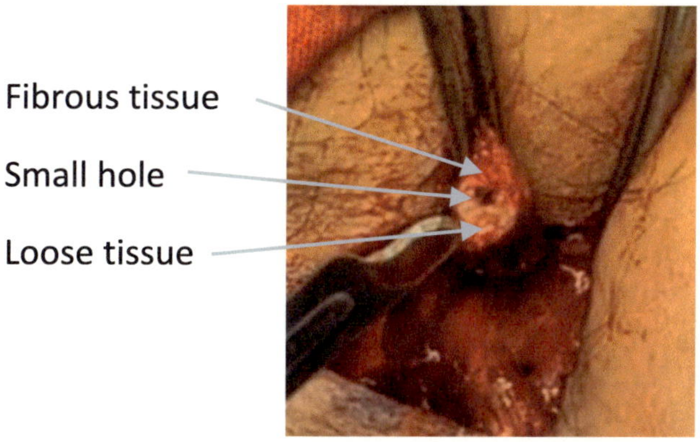

Figure 8.
Recently occluded axillary vein; in AVF repair; you can see that there is a small hole.

Or in case you need open surgery to pass the catheter, a surgeon's help is required.

3. Step-by-step explanation of the procedure

3.1 First step

Perform antisepsis, and surgical fields are placed as for any surgery in the areas that the surgeon considers (**Figure 9**).

3.2 Second step

Puncture of the occluded vein guided by doppler ultrasound and positioning of the guide wire (**Figure 10**).

I prefer to puncture the vein in a place where it is as straight as possible to be able to pass the guide.

That is to say, I prefer to puncture the vein in the right internal jugular vein and both femoral veins, the left subclavian and jugular vein, we have the innominate

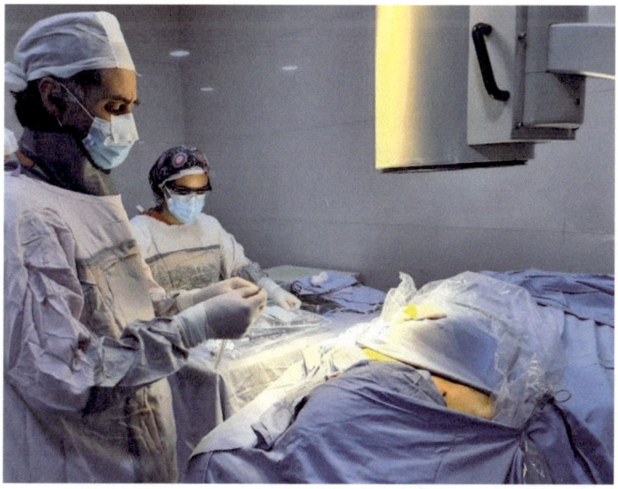

Figure 9.
All set to start, surgical drapes, fluoroscopy, and doppler ultrasound.

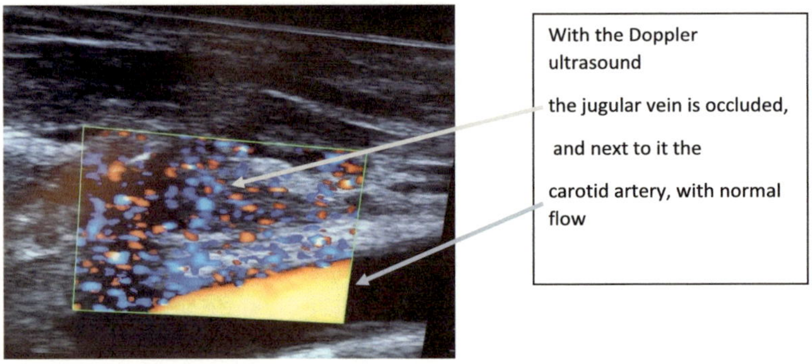

Figure 10.
Doppler photo showing occlusion of the jugular above and orange carotid arterial flow below.

vein curve, and for the right subcalvia a curve of almost 90 degrees to enter the cava.

3.3 Third step

Introduce the needle guided by ultrasound, until it is certain that it is inside the vessel in the middle of the thrombosis. Then introduce a guide wire. Also this has to be verified by ultrasound (**Figure 11**).

3.4 Fourth step

Continue the progression of the guidewire under fluoroscopic control, testing the different types of guidewires, depending on the experience of the operator. In this step, it always helps to advance the guidewire with fine dilators.

It also helped me by injecting contrast to see that anatomically we are in the. correct direction inside the thrombosed vessel (**Figures 12–14**).

3.5 Fifth step

Once the guidewire is sent into the superior or inferior vena cava, and there are no more obstacles, gradually thicker dilators are advanced (**Figure 15**).

3.6 Sixth step

The dilator is inserted with the sheath that corresponds to each catheter. Depending on the case, a double lumen catheter or two catheters are used.

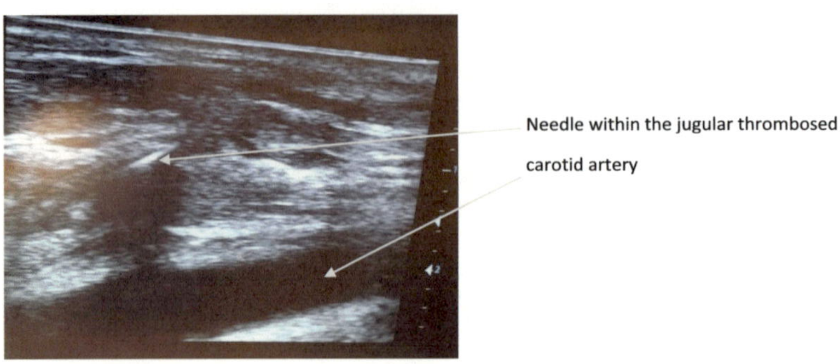

Figure 11.
Photo without doppler shows the needle inside the thrombosed jugular.

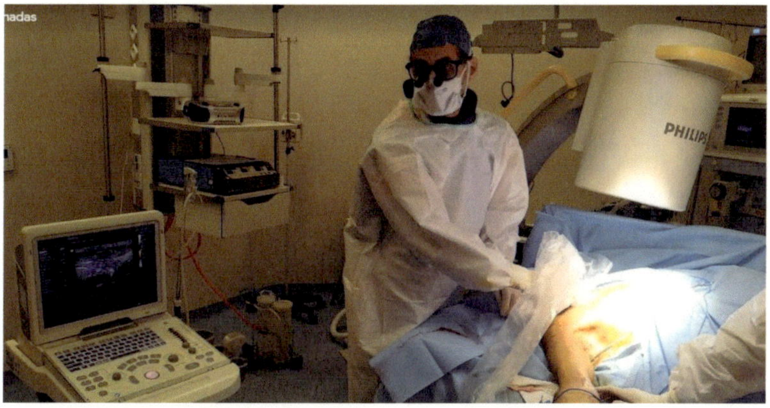

Figure 12.
Looking at the guidewire by doppler ultrasound and fluoroscopy at the same time.

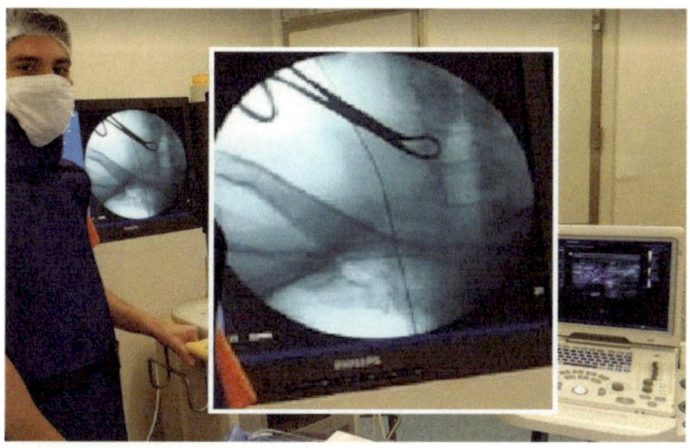

Figure 13.
The guidewire inside superior cava, arrows.

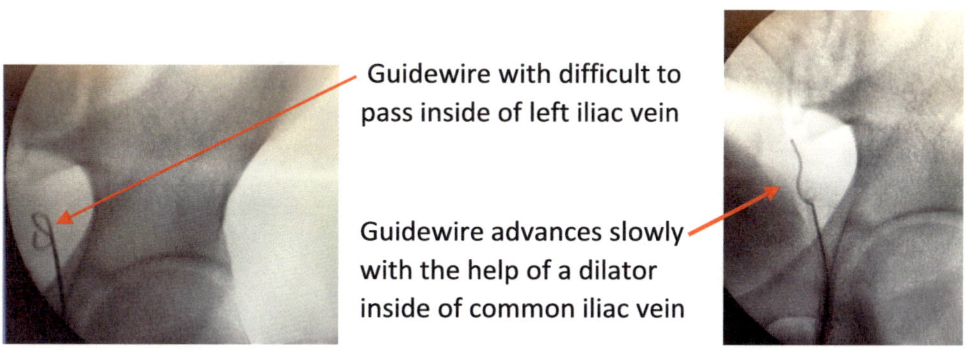

Figure 14.
Guidewire advances through the thrombosed iliac vein.

It can happen that the catheters do not progress through the sheaths, because the strictures are very rigid.

In that case I used thinner catheters inside the haemodialysis catheter. This step can be very cumbersome; so you also have to take it easy and use all your resources and skills to get the catheter where it needs to go (**Figures 16** and **17**).

Some brands of catheter brings thinner semi-rigid catheters for these cases, and they are inserted with 2 guide wires and 2 semi-rigid catheters, one for each lumen (**Figure 18**).

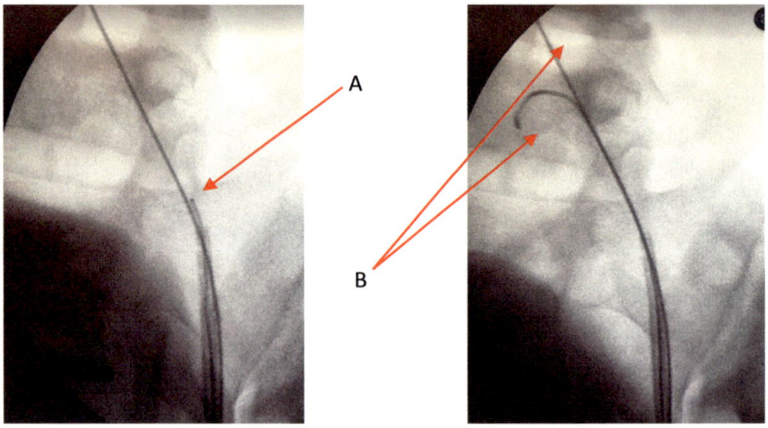

Figure 15.
A Once the guidewire is in the inferior vena cava, in this case, progressively thicker dilators are advanced B Sheath where 2 guide wires were passed.

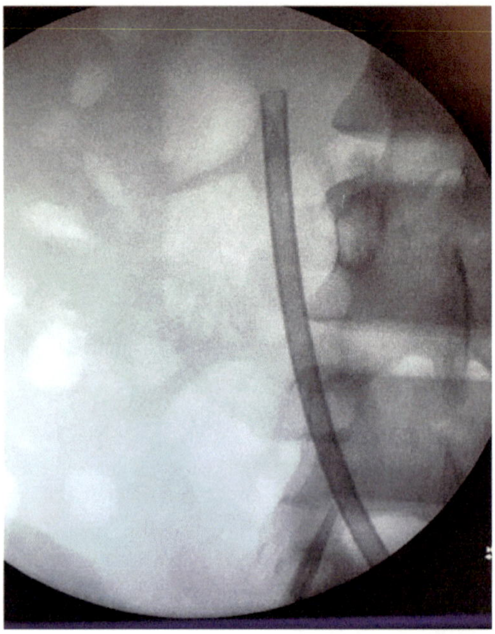

Figure 16.
Double lumen catheter in inferior cava.

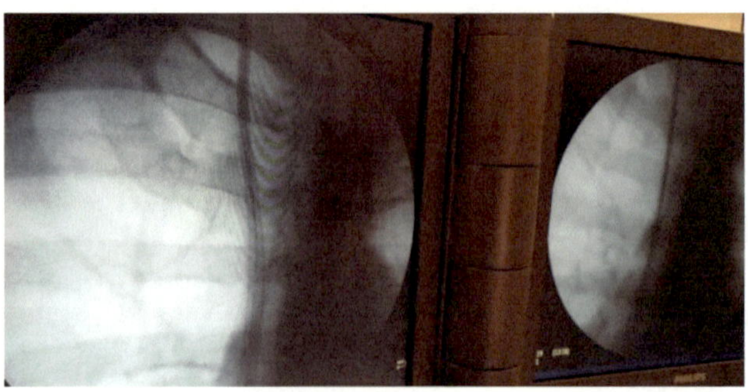

Figure 17.
Double lumen catheter in right atrium by superior cava.

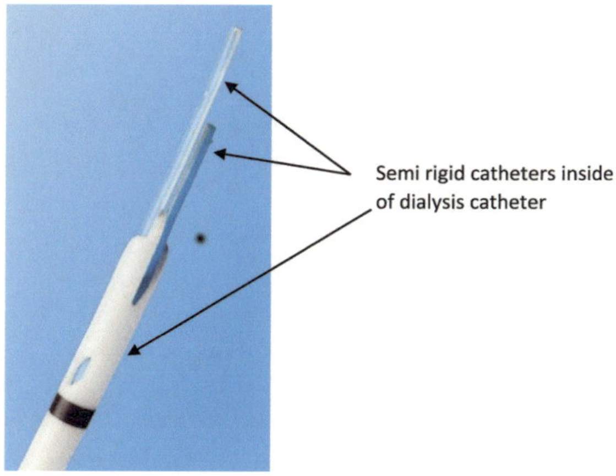

Figure 18.
Catheter model with 2 semi-rigid catheters, which guide wires are passed inside, all this inside the 14 French double lumen catheter.

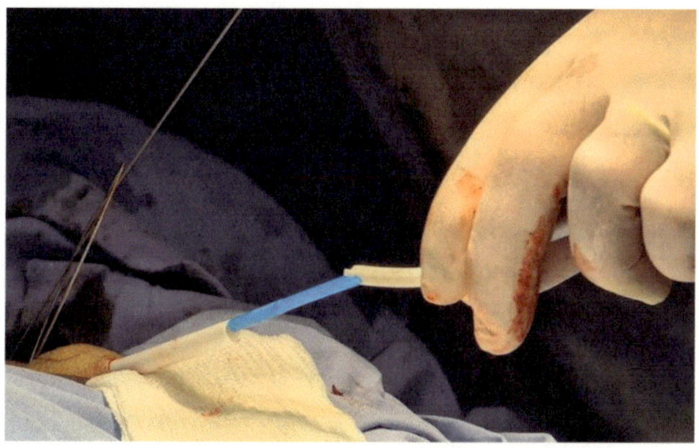

Figure 19.
Tunnelling a double lumen catheter.

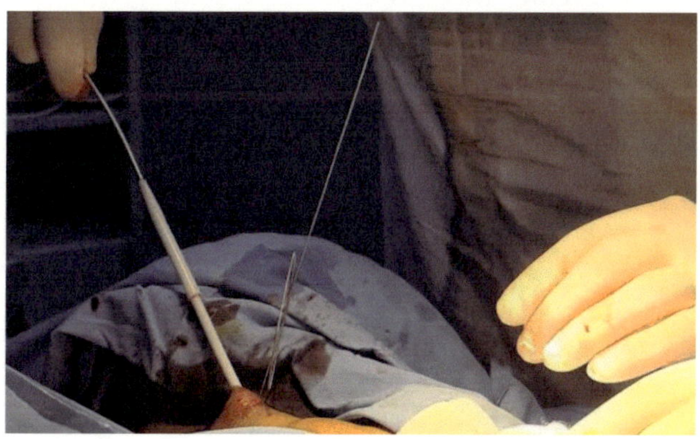

Figure 20.
Tunnelling a double lumen catheter.

3.7 Seventh step

The catheter is positioned and the corresponding tests are performed to obtain adequate flow; tunnelling is performed (**Figures 19–21**).

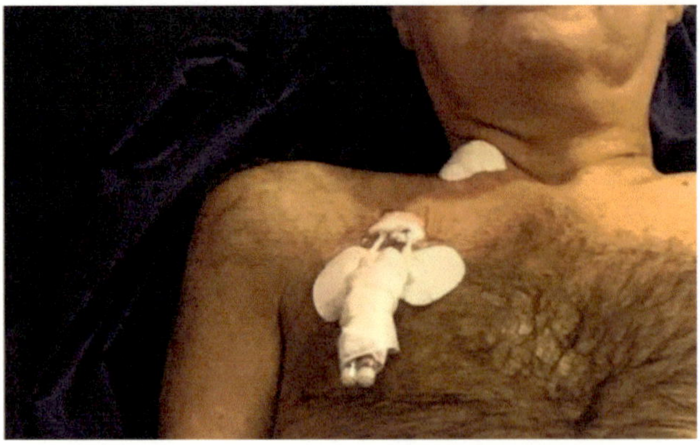

Figure 21.
In this case, we passed the kit of two catheters through the right jugular.

More adequate tunnelling, either with a tunneller that comes with the kit, or with an incision of the necessary size, since some catheters must first be tunnelled and then inserted; this is not possible in these cases because you have to push directly and not through a tunnel.

4. Continue with dialysis

In this way, we can continue with dialysis on these patients, and it gives us time to perform an arteriovenous fistula somewhere.

5. Conclusion

It is not a quick procedure; it requires a lot of patience, previous planning, especially, questioning the patient about his history of vascular access, a meticulous physical examination, and rigorous examination with echo doppler.

Currently, we have several patients operated in this way; I consider it an acceptable technique to save lives with a procedure that until now has had no complications.

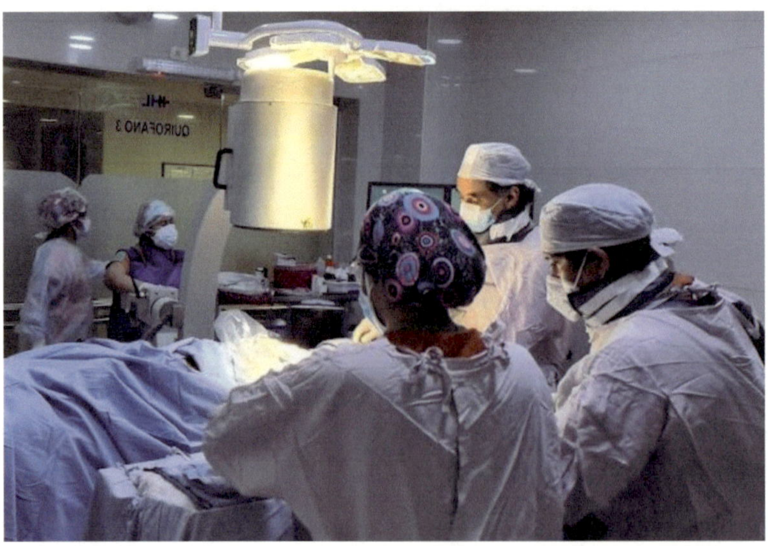

Acknowledgements

To my Family who support me many and many hours in the operating room.
To my colleagues who trust their patients in my hands.
To patients who trust their lives in our hands.

Conflict of interest

The authors declare no conflict of interest.

Notes

All images are my property.

Author details

Arturo Rafael Vizcarra
Scire Cardiovascular SRL, Larcade Hospital, San Miguel, Buenos Aires, Argentina

*Address all correspondence to: avizcarra2@gmail.com

References

[1] Scher LA, Shariff S. Strategies for hemodialysis access: A vascular surgeon's perspective. Techniques in Vascular and Interventional Radiology. 2017;**20**(1):14-19. DOI: 10.1053/j.tvir.2016.11.002

[2] Su SH. Points to remember: Cardiovascular consequences of hemodialysis vascular accesses. Methodist DeBakey Cardiovascular Journal. 2014;**10**(3):202-203. DOI: 10.14797/mdcj-10-3-202.PMID

[3] Loskutov A, Dave A, Gooden C, Saucier NA, Cho KH, Wible BC, et al. Vascular access via translumbar hemodialysis reliable outflow dialysis catheter in a case of severe central venous occlusion. Journal of Vascular Access. 2018;**19**(4):410-411. DOI: 10.1177/1129729818762972

[4] Inston N, Khawaja A, Mistry H, Jones R, Valenti D. Options for end stage vascular access: Translumbar catheter, arterial-arterial access or right atrial graft? Journal of Vascular Access. 2020;**21**(1):7-18. DOI: 10.1177/1129729819841153

[5] Jeffrey HL, Niklason LE, Roy-Chaudhury P. Challenges and novel therapies for vascular access in haemodialysis. Nature Reviews Nephrology. 2020;**16**:586-602

[6] Gouda ZE, Emara MM, Elbarbary HS, Koura MAA, Elarbagy AR. Studying alternative approaches for placement of cuffed hemodialysis catheters in hemodialysis patients with bilateral internal jugular vein occlusion. Journal of Vascular Access. 2019;**20**(3):250-259. DOI: 10.1177/1129729818794414

[7] Vizcarra A, Hermida O. Exhaustion of vascular accesses for hemodialysis: access by thrombosed vein. Revista de Nefrología, Diálisis y Trasplante. 2020;**40**(02):179-182

Chapter 5

Patient Safety in Hemodialysis

Renata De Paula Faria Rocha

Abstract

Patient safety addresses the risks involved in health care, simplifying or eliminating adverse events, these are defined as incidents that occur during the provision of health care and that result in harm to the patient. Health care is increasingly complex and can increase the potential for incidents, errors or failures to occur. Hemodialysis is a technically complex procedure, with many potential sources of error and which can cause harm to patients. Dialysis is a therapy that in recent years has benefited many patients, but it is a care process that involves important dangers and risks. Hemodialysis is a hospital sector with a great risk potential for the occurrence of adverse events, this occurs for several reasons such as complex procedures, the use of high technology, the characteristic of chronic kidney disease, the high use of medications. Strategies need to be taken to reduce the occurrence of adverse events, thus ensuring the quality of dialysis, consequently the quality of life of patients with chronic kidney disease undergoing dialysis treatment.

Keywords: renal dialysis, patient safety, nursing care, chronic renal failure, nursing in nephrology

1. Introduction

Patient safety is defined by the World Health Organization (WHO) as reducing the risk of unnecessary harm associated with healthcare to an acceptable minimum [1].

The topic of patient safety has been increasingly disseminated within institutions and among healthcare professionals, about the search for the quality of care provided and the reduction of preventable incidents [2].

Patient safety addresses the risks involved in health care to reduce or eliminate Adverse Events (AEs), defined as incidents that occur during health care and result in harm to the patient, characterized as physical, social, and psychological, including illness, injury, suffering, disability or death [1].

The interest in this topic is a result of the realization that the occurrence of Adverse Events (AEs) involves considerable social and economic costs, and may involve irreversible damage to patients and their families [3].

The patient safety issue began with the publication of the Institute of Medicine (IOM) report To Err is Human. This publication provoked the mobilization of the medical class and the public in general, of North American organizations and several countries for issues related to patient safety. This mobilization is the result of the realization that the occurrence of adverse events (AE) involves considerable social and economic costs, and can cause irreversible damage to patients and their families. The IOM report estimated the occurrence of 44 to 98 thousand deaths each year, in the United States (USA), resulting from AEs [4].

IntechOpen

According to the Institute of Medicine (1999) quality in healthcare, considering current scientific knowledge, is defined as the degree to which the services provided to the patient, on the one hand, decrease the probability of unfavorable outcomes, and, on the other, increase the probability of favorable outcomes. Unfavorable outcomes are adverse events (AEs).

Developments in patient safety and reliability of health services imply a change in the conduct practiced by most services. The safety culture of an organization is the set of values, attitudes, perceptions, competencies, and behavioral patterns that determine the commitment, style, and proficiency of the administration of a healthcare organization with safety management [5].

Health care is increasingly complex, and predisposes the occurrence of incidents, errors or failures. Injuries or damage resulting from the care provided constitute a serious problem related to the performance of health services; unsafe health care can cause increased morbidity and mortality worldwide [6].

Researches that investigate the patient safety culture in the hospital environment are increasingly present in the scientific environment. The positive safety culture favors the improvement of safe practices, through improvements in communication, teamwork and knowledge sharing [3].

The development of a safety culture, the practice of records, the discussion about the circumstances in which incidents occur, as well as the professional and organizational behaviors in front of this situation, constitute a path to be followed for the transformation of the reality in health institutions [7].

In this perspective, the development of safety culture has received increasing attention in the field of healthcare organizations. The complexity present in health care, which involves its dynamic and multifaceted nature, the use of leading-edge technology and the action of professionals from different fields, predisposes to error and, to minimize it, potential sources must be identified and prioritized [8].

It is a fact that unsafe health care can result in increased morbidity and mortality, which makes this a global concern, because many errors could be avoidable from the implementation of safety indicators in quality monitoring programs in the care offered to hospitalized patients [9].

It is currently recommended that, in assessing the impact of events related to patient safety, not only mortality but also morbidity be considered given the repercussions on the quality of life of patients who have suffered damage [5].

Chronic kidney disease (CKD) is a condition with several attributes that have the potential to increase the risk of errors and patient safety failures. People with CKD have higher rates of hospitalizations, which leaves them susceptible to interventions with the potential for errors to occur [10].

There is a high proportion of people with chronic kidney disease (CKD) who experience safety-related events. This factor highlights the vulnerability of this population to potential adverse effects of care [11].

Patients with CKD have hemodialysis as one of the treatment modalities. Regarding the Hemodialysis Service, it is emphasized that the treatment is complex, with specific activities, for example, the control of the extracorporeal blood circulation system, requiring adequate structure and trained professionals for a safe care practice, which, if not respected, may cause irreversible damage to the user [12].

Hemodialysis (HD) is a technically complex procedure, with many potential sources of error that can cause harm to patients. Carrying out hemodialysis safely requires many steps, ranging from creating the dialyzer and other equipment, accessing the bloodstream and monitoring the patient to prevent complications and ensure hemodynamic stability [13].

Dialysis is a therapy that in recent years has been benefiting many patients, but it is a care process that involves important dangers and risks. The risks of hemodialysis in situations of chronic disease comorbidities are related to the fact that the patient has a terminal disease that depends on permanent life support, in addition to the use of many medications [5].

The complexity of hemodialysis procedures specifically involves the use of advanced technologies, water quality, dialyser reuse, infection control, machine disinfection and the use of medications [8]. The complexity of chronic kidney disease (CKD): the chronicity of the disease, the involvement of multiple health care professionals, and the different activities of care [14].

Thus, in this type of procedure, considering the frequency with which patients undergo the procedure that involves the use of high technology, it is important to evaluate issues related to patient safety.

There are several risk factors for adverse events in hemodialysis, among which he highlights: invasive procedures, use of complex equipment, critical patients, high patient turnover, and administration of potentially dangerous drugs such as heparin [15].

The authors conducted a study in which they identified some avoidable variables that may have contributed to the deaths of patients on hemodialysis. They point out that these variables were related to communication, organization, and human factors, associated with five main causes, for example: the treatment of hyperkalemia, the prescription, the time of treatment, the presence of infection, and vascular access [16].

The use of Checklists is a patient safety strategy that can be effective. Checklists are tools used to improve patient safety, adherence to protocols and policies, contribute to communication, teamwork, and the standardization of procedures [17].

Authors emphasize that the use of Checklists is an important strategy to ensure that procedures are performed safely, as it allows the occurrence/recurrence of preventable harm to be identified and prevented [13].

When used properly, guidelines, protocols, and checklists can result in quality care, considerably reducing the risks presented by the procedures to which the patient has been submitted.

Checklists were initially used in surgical and intensive care environments and have been shown to be an important patient safety strategy that can improve the safety culture [18].

High-quality institutions with a good safety culture anticipate adverse events as a way to prepare professionals to deal with them at all levels of the organization. In this way, they make tools available to professionals to develop skills to convert such adverse events into improved system resistance [19].

Patient safety assessment enables hospitals to prospectively identify and manage relevant safety issues in their work routines [20].

Care for patients receiving renal replacement therapy (RRT) is complex and technology dependent; patients have a high burden of comorbidity, polypharmacy, and the physiological consequences of established kidney disease means that patients on RRT are potentially vulnerable to errors [16].

Patient safety events can have costly consequences for patients and healthcare networks, increasing length of stay, readmissions to the hospital, and the risk of death [11].

Hemodialysis units are sites susceptible to the occurrence of adverse events (AE) because they have several risk factors, such as invasive procedures, use of complex equipment, water treatment, critical patients, high patient turnover and administration of potentially dangerous drugs, such as heparin. A study performed in four hemodialysis units in the USA identified that in a 17-month period 88 adverse events occurred during 64,541 dialysis treatments (01 case for every 733 treatments) [15].

The presence of infection in the SRT population is a complex and common problem, since the prevalence of sepsis in dialysis patients is more than 100 times higher than the general population, is multifactorial, associated with high hospitalization rates, infection risks, and immunosuppression as a consequence of renal impairment, comorbidity, and immunosuppressive therapy [16].

Bloodstream infections are the main causes of death and hospitalization among hemodialysis patients, in second place are cardiovascular diseases [21].

Among the main causes of AEs in hemodialysis patients, the patient's clinical condition is very important. Such conditions directly influence the occurrence of AEs, especially in critically ill patients, given the hemodynamic instability and the need for interventions, which make them particularly vulnerable to adverse events [22].

In addition, CKD is associated with pathophysiological changes such as anemia, osteopenia, susceptibility to hypervolemia, electrolyte changes and infection, which can increase the risk of complications and adverse events [10].

For the occurrence of AEs, there are psychological and physiological factors that can influence the behavior of professionals during care and interfere with patient safety [22].

In daily nursing care, it is clear that the number of professionals directly influences the implementation of measures related to the implementation of a culture of safety. Thus, an adequate dimensioning of the team is essential, as it interferes in the administrative process and consequent care planning [22].

About the weekly workload, 48% of nursing professionals in the hemodialysis unit work from 50 to 70 hours per week, increasing the risk of failures being committed during the provision of care. The risks of the professional committing an error increase significantly when the work day exceeds 40 hours per week, when work shifts exceed 12 hours or when overtime is performed [23].

Thus, it can be observed that the working hours and the dimensioning of nursing staff are factors that can interfere in the quality of the care provided, consequently influencing the safety of the patient on hemodialysis.

2. Factors affecting patient safety in hemodialysis

A study aiming to assess the frequency of adverse events occurred in CKD patients, shows that about half of the participants had one or two safety events. Diabetic patients were 2.9 times more likely to have three or four adverse safety events compared to non-diabetic patients. In addition, patients with stage 5 CKD were 2.8 times more likely than patients with stage 3 CKD to have multiple safety events during the study period [11].

These data reinforce the assertion that patients with CKD are more vulnerable to safety failures related to their clinical condition. CKD is a significant risk factor for many safety events.

In the other study, direct complications of CRT accounted for 2.1% of deaths, and 3.5% of deaths of patients on CRT [16].

The Pennsylvania Patient Safety Authority, an independent agency in the United States of America (USA) charged with taking action to reduce and eliminate health care failures, developed a study to understand the types of errors and AEs occurring during hemodialysis. An analysis of 526 reports of events related to hemodialysis treatment over a one-year period was performed. Medication errors were the most prevalent (28.5%), followed by failure to follow protocol (12.9%) [24].

The conditions identified as predisposing to adverse events in hemodialysis patients are: hyperkalemia, hypoglycemia, prescription of medications in a safe manner, the presence of infection, and vascular access for hemodialysis [11, 16].

In dialysis services, hand hygiene is an important infection control measure, since, in this scenario, several patients undergo dialysis treatment at the same time, in the same environment, which can contribute to the spread of microorganisms. This dissemination can occur through direct or indirect contact, through devices, equipment, surfaces or through the hands of health professionals [12].

Central venous catheter infections for hemodialysis are much more frequent when compared to arteriovenous fistulas [21].

Complications associated with vascular access can be severe, causing a high risk of morbidity and mortality for patients. Bloodstream infections represent a major impact on the morbidity and mortality of this population. Nurses must monitor, detect and intervene in complications that occur during hemodialysis sessions [22].

The arteriovenous fistula (AVF) is the most appropriate and safest venous access, because it is the long-standing access that enables effective dialysis with fewer interventions [25].

Thus, the use of double-lumen catheter can lead to a higher occurrence of adverse events, interfering with the safety of the patient on hemodialysis. CDL infection is one of the main adverse events in hemodialysis. The largest number of infections in patients undergoing hemodialysis procedure is related to the Temporary Double Lumen Catheter (TDCL). Bacteremia in patients with a catheter during HD varies from 4–18% and in most cases associated with hyperthemia. Infectious complications are causative agents of increasing morbidity and mortality in hemodialysis patients [26].

CKD is also characterized by impaired renal clearance of numerous medications, increasing the risk for incorrect dosing and toxicity of therapeutic agents [10].

In the hemodialysis community, medication errors are reported as the most common patient safety event. Medication errors are common among dialysis patients and often occur as errors of omission [11, 21].

In addition to medication omission errors, errors also occur during medication administration and communication errors among the team [21].

Obstruction of the venous catheter is a very frequent adverse event in hemodialysis sessions. It occurs when a clot forms in the catheter lumen, preventing blood flow from the patient's body to the hemodialysis machine, which leads to the loss of the blood volume that fills the system [22].

The blood clotting of the extracorporeal system usually occurs in sessions performed without heparin, due to contraindication of the drug [22].

Problems in vascular access that lead to adequate blood flow interfere directly in the dialysis dose, reducing the Kt/V, consequently interfering with the patient's health status.

Events of hyperkalemia and hypoglycemia were found individually, are common adverse events, as well as risk factors for mortality of patients with CKD [11].

In a hemodialysis session, it is necessary to check vital signs to avoid episodes of hypotension, consequently, the cramps, headache and nausea, verification of blood glucose to avoid episodes of hypoglycemia and, plus correct checking and noting of weight and body temperature; anticoagulation, proper functioning of the dialysis machines (temperature, roller, blood flow, dialysate flow), being important the use of a checklist to avoid negligence.

Failure to comply with this verification routine is considered negligence, which is an action diverging from the correct one, arising from the professional's passivity or omission, which can lead to episodes of hypotension, hypoglycemia, among others, thus configuring the occurrence of an adverse event [25].

Accidental removal of the needle that punctures the arteriovenous fistula can be considered one of the most dangerous AEs in hemodialysis units, as the patient can bleed to death in a few minutes. Therefore, it is necessary for nursing to adopt measures that reduce the risk of this event occurring [22].

Infiltration of the hemodialysis access and coagulation of the hemodialysis circuit are some adverse events that can occur.

About dialysis programming, one can highlight the definition of the dry weight, the kt/v and the programming of the parameters in the dialysis machine.

The quality of the dialysis offered to the patients can be measured by the Kt/V. The Kt/V represents the adequacy of dialysis. In this study, it is observed that there is no record of Kt/V in 94% of the analyzed medical records.

There is a correlation between hemodialysis (HD) dose and patient morbidity and mortality, so to estimate whether CKD patients on HD receive adequate treatment, the HD dose should be measured. Clinical signs and symptoms are very important, but they are not sufficient indicators of dialysis dose [27].

Kt/V assessment is nursing care and refers to providing quality dialysis to the patient. There are several factors related to achieving an ideal Kt/V, and it is important to emphasize that the patient needs to adhere to the treatment as recommended, i.e., perform the dialysis time, follow the diets, take medications, take care of the vascular access.

The other part is up to the multidisciplinary team, which includes providing guidance. The dialysis service must be committed to the treatment, offering an ideal capillary according to the body mass, performing good venous access, correct adequacy during treatment [28].

The National Kidney Foundation considers the ideal hemodialysis dose a Kt/V greater than 1.2, for the patient who performs hemodialysis three times a week and for four hours each session [28].

Incorrect programming is an adverse event and can lead to significant losses to the patient, even death.

Checking the schedule is the nurse's role, since this is the professional of the health team responsible for managing care in dialysis units. Nursing in hemodialysis treatment has great relevance regarding the uninterrupted observation of patients during the period in which the hemodialysis session occurs [29].

In the Renal Physicians Association survey, 17 percent of patients indicated that they had problems with the settings on their dialysis machines. In this study, the authors point out that patients involved in their dialysis care are significantly less likely to report having had problems with machine settings [30].

Dry weight is the target weight to be achieved post hemodialysis below which all, or most of the excess fluid has been removed, without developing symptoms of hypotension [25].

Adherence to adequate fluid intake is commonly measured by interdialytic weight gain (GPID). The adequate dry weight prevents the occurrence of hypotension or hypertension.

Studies have shown a relationship between elevated GPID and complications such as hypertension, congestive heart failure, and even death. In addition, the removal of this excess fluid during hemodialysis (HD) can result in episodes of hypotension, muscle cramps, nausea, and headache [31].

The nurse has a fundamental role as an educator, providing the necessary guidance for patients to maintain their interdialytic weight gain within the recommended values.

Adherence to dietary and fluid restrictions improves laboratory parameters, reduces complications such as hospitalizations for acute pulmonary edema and improves the quality of life of patients on HD [32].

The conventional treatment regimen of three sessions per week implies long periods without hemodialysis, especially on weekends, when the patient can consume a larger amount of fluids and not follow the diet as he should. Thus, there is an oscillation in the volume of liquids and biochemistry during the following week, where it is possible to observe an increase in complications in the sessions at the beginning of the week. The ideal would be more frequent or longer sessions, to offer more security and increase the life expectancy of these patients [33].

The mechanicity present in hemodialysis treatment leads professionals to present a posture of "doing for doing", which lends to the activities a feeling of accommodation, which is summarized in, every shift, putting the patient on the machine, pushing the button and supervising its operation [34].

Nursing in nephrology is specialized care, but the nursing action should not be reduced to the performance of a set of techniques. In HD, it is necessary to provide care based on the training of professionals to seek the best conditions to provide quality of life for the patient. Therefore, nursing care in this scenario also involves interactive action, supported by the ethical dimension between the one who cares and the one who is cared for [35].

3. Strategies for patient safety in hemodialysis

Patient safety deals with the risks involved in health care and seeks to minimize these risks and reduce or eliminate Adverse Events, which are incidents that result in harm to the patient [1].

Preventing adverse events can improve the quality of care and patient outcomes [11].

Quality comprises the relentless search for identifying flaws in procedures and practices that organize actions, leading to improved processes and results, aiming at the conformities established by regulatory agencies and user satisfaction [12].

Reducing errors and improving patient safety have become a national priority. Patients with chronic kidney disease (CKD) may be at higher risk for adverse consequences of medical care, but few studies have evaluated this issue [10].

The occurrence of AEs can be minimized by changing managerial and professional attitudes, strengthening leadership, improving access to information, quality, maintenance and use of equipment and environments as well as knowledge and encouraging continuing education [7].

Safety culture has received increasing attention in the field of healthcare organizations. Healthcare is becoming increasingly complex, raising the potential for incidents, errors, or failures to occur. Injuries or harm resulting from the care provided are a serious problem related to the performance of health services; unsafe health care causes significant morbidity and mortality worldwide [6].

From this perspective, health institutions must develop strategies for a patient safety culture. The development of protocols that standardize procedures makes the work process safer and more efficient [22].

Professionals should have knowledge about adverse events and their impact on health care, since the incidence of these events is an important indicator of quality [22].

Currently, there is a greater awareness, nationwide, that professionals need to be trained about the measures to be taken in case of failures, in addition to being encouraged to take an honest attitude towards the error, without fear of punishment and effectively involved in the search for safe patient care [36].

Nursing professionals are responsible for most of the care actions and, therefore, are in a privileged position to reduce the possibility of incidents affecting the patient, as well as to detect complications early and perform the necessary procedures to minimize damage [22].

The maintenance of good adequacy of hemodialysis in patients with chronic kidney disease depends directly on an efficient Vascular Access (VA), whose complications have great representativeness among the morbidities in this group. And, considering the importance of the VA, it is worth noting that the effectiveness of therapy is closely associated with its implantation, handling and proper monitoring, affecting the quality of dialysis and, consequently, the well-being and survival of the patient [12].

Adverse events related to vascular access can be avoided using improvements in the care processes used by Nursing, as well as constant evaluation of the results of the practices adopted.

Studies show that catheter-related infections can be reduced when prevention measures are properly applied, such as the use of aseptic technique before insertion, in each manipulation of the device and dressings, antisepsis at the catheter exit site with 2% alcoholic chlorhexidine, adequate staff paramentation (sterile gloves, masks, goggles and aprons), care in catheter maintenance, monitoring of infection signs, continuing education of staff professionals and self-care guidance for the patient [37, 38].

Considering that vascular accesses are an important care practice and are closely related to the quality of care and quality of life of CKD patients, it is believed that the use of checklists can be an important ally in the evaluation of vascular access, ensuring the quality of this therapeutic modality [22, 39].

The Nursing team that works in hemodialysis units must have knowledge about adverse events to be able to identify the risks and the situations that favor their occurrence, to seek alternatives to minimize failures, adopt risk analysis methods and thus ensure the quality of the services [22].

Many hospitalizations may be preventable with better care planning, adequate patient education, and early detection of complications [40].

Strategies to improve patient safety in dialysis units have emphasized the importance of effective communication, reduction of medication errors, correct dialysis, equipment preparation, and infection control [16].

Encouraging the practice of hand hygiene constitutes one of the nine solutions for patient safety, launched in 2007, in the Nine Patient Safety Solutions program, considered the primary preventive measure to avoid harm to patients [12].

The Nine Patient Safety Solutions program is based on patient safety strategies and best practices that have been identified by the WHO World Alliance for Patient Safety. They were developed with feedback from more than 50 patient safety experts from over 100 countries. The strategies come in nine titles and are being made available to WHO member states. The intention is that the strategies will be used to reexamine patient care processes to improve safety [1].

The nine points covered by the program are: Identical medication names; Patient identification; Communication; Correct procedure in the correct place; Control of concentrated electrolyte solutions; Medication accuracy; Care with connections; Single-use of injection and hand hygiene devices [1].

The theme described above is recurrent in health services and treated as a priority by programs and initiatives that focus on safety in patient care, such as the World Alliance for Patient Safety, an initiative of the WHO, which has dedicated efforts in the development of guidelines and strategies for implementation of measures, including adherence to the practice of hand hygiene and, more recently, in Brazil, by the Ordinance of the Ministry of Health No. 529/2013, which establishes the National Program for Patient Safety [41].

Organizations must safely structure the system, helping professionals not to make mistakes. All causes should be analyzed by the risk management service for the development of corrective actions, aiming at the prevention and reduction of adverse events [22].

Among the suggestions to prevent the occurrence of adverse events, continuing education was mentioned as the main measure and as an important action for human resource training and development. The nursing staff of a hemodialysis unit should develop skills to detect and prevent adverse events, adopting strategies to improve the care processes developed in daily practice [22].

Health education can also contribute to patient safety. A good level of understanding of the disease and treatment aspects also positively influences the patient's adaptation and adherence to treatment [42].

This factor could reflect a lower occurrence of adverse events related to hemodialysis treatment.

Dialysis centers must function as high-reliability organizations to improve patient safety. These services must establish a culture of safety, which is based on communication based on mutual trust, common perceptions about the importance of safety and confidence in the effectiveness of preventive measures [21].

In the occurrence of an incident, what is important is the assimilation that the cause of errors and adverse events is multifactorial and that healthcare professionals are susceptible to committing them when technical and organizational processes are complex and poorly planned [22].

The high frequency of different events observed reveals the specialized care needs for the CKD population. Providing safe care for this population, therefore, provides some unique challenges.

Research must advance in understanding the cause of harm, identifying solutions, impact, and transposing evidence to the organization of care. They reinforce that measuring harm is fundamental to know the patient safety problem [43].

Author details

Renata De Paula Faria Rocha
Centro Universitário de Brasília–CEUB, Brazil

*Address all correspondence to: rpfrocha@gmail.com

References

[1] World Health Organization (WHO). Global Priorities for Patient Safety Research. Switzerland, Geneva; 2009. Available from: http://www.who.int/patientsafety/research/priorities

[2] Lorenzini E, Santi JAR, Báo ACP. Segurança do paciente: Análise dos incidentes notificados em um hospital do sul do Brasil. Revista Gaúcha de Enfermagem. 2014;**35**(2):121-127

[3] Reis CT, Martins M, Laguardia J. A segurança do paciente como dimensão da qualidade do cuidado de saúde – um olhar sobre a literatura. Ciências de Saúde Coletiva. 2013;**18**(7):2029-2036

[4] Kohn LT, Corrigan JM, Donaldson MC, Committee on Quality of Health Care; Institute of Medicine. To Err is Human: Building a Safer Health System. Washington (DC): National Academy Press; 2000

[5] Vieira C, Silva DR, Prates CG. Segurança do paciente em serviços de diálise. São Paulo: Livraria Balieira; 2019

[6] Reis CT, Laguardia J, Martins M. Adaptação transcultural da versão brasileira do Hospital Survey on Patient Safety Culture: etapa inicial. Cadernos de Saúde Pública. 2012;**28**(11):2199-2210

[7] Paranaguá TTB et al. Prevalence of no harm incidents and adverse events in a surgical clinic. Acta Paulista de Enfermagem. 2013;**26**(3):256-262

[8] Garrick R, Kliger A, Stefanchik B. Patient and facility safety in hemodialysis: Opportunities and strategies to develop a culture of safety. Clinical Journal of the American Society of Nephrology. 2012;**7**:680-688

[9] Gouvea CSD, Travassos C. Indicadores de segurança do paciente para hospitais de pacientes agudos: revisão sistemática. Cadernos de Saúde Pública. 2010;**26**(6):1061-1078

[10] Seliger SL et al. Chronic kidney disease Adversely influences patient safety. American Society of Nephrology. 2008;**19**:2414-2419

[11] Chapin et al. Safety events in chronic kidney disease: The frequency of "Multiple Hits". Clinical Journal of the American Society of Nephrology. 2010;**5**:95-101

[12] Rich NC et al. A mixed-methods investigation of incident hemodialysis access in a safety-net population. BMC Nephrology. 2017;**18**:279

[13] Bray BD, Metcalfe W. Improving patient safety in haemodialysis. Clinical Kidney Journal. 2015;**8**:262-264

[14] Van Der Veer S et al. Translating knowledge on best practice into improving quality of RRT care: A systematic review of implementation strategies. Kidney International. 2011;**80**:1021-1034

[15] Holley JL. A descripve report of errors and adverse events in chronic hemodialysis units. Nephrology News & Issues. 2006;**20**(12):57-63

[16] Bray BD et al. How safe is renal replacement therapy? A national study of mortality and adverse events contributing to the death of renal replacement therapy recipients. Nephrology, Dialysis, Transplantation. 2014;**29**:681-687

[17] Silver SA et al. Development of a hemodialysis safety checklist using a structured panel process. Canadian Journal of Kidney Health and Disease. 2015;**2**:5

[18] Treadwel JR, Lucas S, Tsou AY. Surgical checklists: A systematic review of impacts and implementation. BMJ Quality and Safety. 2014;**23**:299-318

[19] Lima FDM. A segurança do paciente e intervenções para a qualidade dos

cuidados de saúde. Revista Espaço Para a Saúde. 2014;**15**(3):22-29

[20] Sorra JS, Nieva VF. Hospital Survey on Patient Safety Culture. Rockville: Agency for Healthcare Research and Quality; 2004

[21] Kliger AS. Maintaining safety in the dialysis facility. Clinical Journal of the American Society of Nephrology. 2015;**10**:688-695

[22] Thomas A et al. Feasibility of a hemodialysis safety checklist for nurses and patients: A quality improvement study. Clinical Kidney Journal. 2016;**9**(3):335-342

[23] Duarte SCM et al. Eventos adversos e segurança na assistência de enfermagem. Revista Brasileira de Enfermagem. 2015;**68**(1):144-154

[24] Pennsylvania Patient Safety Authority. Hemodialysis administration: Strategies to ensure safe patient care. Pennsylvania Patient Safety Advisory. 2010;**7**(3):87-97. Available from: http://patientsafetyauthority.org/ADVISORIES/AdvisoryLibrary/2010/Sep7%283%29/documents/87.pdf

[25] Daugirdas JT, Blake PG, Ing TS. Manual de diálise. 5ª ed. Rio de Janeiro: Guanabara Koogan; 2016

[26] Terra FS et al. As principais complicações apresentadas pelos pacientes renais crônicos durante as sessões de hemodiálise. Revista da Sociedade Brasileira de Clínica Médica. 2010;**8**(3):187-192

[27] Breitsameter G, Figueiredo AE, Kochhann DS. Cálculo de Kt/V em hemodiálise: comparação entre fórmulas. Jornal Brasileiro de Nefrologia. 2012;**34**(1):22-26

[28] National Kidney Foundation (NKF). Updates Clinical Practice Guidelines and Recommendations. New York: EUA; 2006

[29] Rocha MTFB et al. O Papel da Enfermagem na Sessão de Hemodiálise. Revista Científica Multidisciplinar Núcleo do Conhecimento. Edição Especial de Saúde. 2017;**2**(4):39-52

[30] Renal Physicians Association, 2007. https://www.renalmd.org/

[31] Smith K et al. Patient perspectives on fluid management in chronic hemodialysis. Journal of Renal Nutrition. 2010;**20**:331-341

[32] Nerbass FB et al. Fatores relacionados ao ganho de peso interdialítico em pacientes em hemodiálise. Jornal Brasileiro de Nefrologia. 2011;**33**(3):300-305

[33] Matos JPS, Lugon JR. Alternative hemodialysis regimens. Jornal Brasileiro de Nefrologia. 2010;**32**(1):114-119

[34] Willig MH, Lenardt MH, Trentini M. Gerenciamento e cuidado em Unidades de Hemodiálise. Revista Brasileira de Enfermagem. 2006;**59**(2): 177-182

[35] Martins MRI, Cesarino CB. Qualidade de vida de pessoas com insuficiência renal crônica em tratamento hemodialítico. Revista Latino-Americana de Enfermagem. 2005;**13**(5):670-676

[36] Leitão IMTA et al. Análise da comunicação de eventos adversos na perspectiva de enfermeiros assistenciais. Rev Rene. 2013;**14**(6):1073-1083

[37] Schwanke AA. Fatores de risco associados à infecção em cateter venoso central para hemodiálise. 91f. [Dissertação (Mestrado)]. In: apresentada ao Programa de Pós-graduação em Enfermagem da Universidade Federal do Paraná. Brasil: Curitiba. 2016

[38] Fram DS et al. Prevenção de infecções de corrente sanguínea

relacionadas a cateter em pacientes em hemodiálise. Acta Paulista de Enfermagem. 2009;**22**(2):564-568

[39] Nicole AG, Tronchin DMR. Indicadores para avaliação do acesso vascular de usuários em hemodiálise. Revista da Escola de Enfermagem da U.S.P. 2011;**45**(1):206-214

[40] Thomas-Hawkins C et al. Nurse manager safety practices in out patient hemodialysis units. Nephrology Nursing Journal. 2015;**42**(2):125-133

[41] Arenas MD et al. A multicentric survey of the practice of hand hygiene in haemodialysis units: Factors affecting compliance. Nephrology, Dialysis, Transplantation. 2005;**20**:1164-1171

[42] Freitas PPW, Cosmo M. Atuação do Psicólogo em Hemodiálise. Revista da Sociedade Brasileira de Psicologia Hospitalar. 2010;**13**(1):19-32

[43] Martins M, Mendes W. Cuidado seguro: um desafio a mais para as organizações de saúde. Cadernos de Saúde Pública. 2016;**32**(10):e00160516

Section 3

Renal-Associated Diseases and Clinical Biomarkers

Chapter 6

Specific Cerebrovascular Risk Factors, Colon Microbiocenosis and Its Correction in Patients Receiving Long-Term Programmed Hemodialysis

Alexey E. Khrulev, Irina V. Belova, Irina V. Soloveva, Anna G. Tochilina, Natalya A. Shiyanova, Anastasiya A. Nikitina and Natalya S. Khruleva

Abstract

Introduction: The problem of acute and chronic cerebrovascular disorders in dialysis patients remains the most urgent. Risk factors for cerebrovascular diseases in CKD and dialysis patients can be conditionally divided into "*traditional*" (arterial hypertension, diabetes mellitus, hypercholesterolemia) and "*specific*" (associated with renal pathology and dialysis procedures). The spectrum of specific factors of cerebrovascular risk in patients with dialysis stage of the CKD includes specific dialysis factors that form during programmed HD, as well as impaired phosphorus-calcium metabolism and calcification of the arterial microvasculature, increased blood levels of β2-microglobulin, homocysteine, malondialdehyde and superoxide dismutase, a decrease in the level of nitric oxide (II) metabolites, development of nephrogenic anemia and dysfunction of blood cells, malnutrition and dietary features of patients with renal pathology, accumulation of uremic toxins and toxins of intestinal bacteria, etc. Opportunistic gut microorganisms can produce uremic toxins, which are associated with an increased risk of inflammation, increased oxidative stress, and a higher risk of cardiovascular disease (CVD). Description of the spectrum of risk factors for cerebrovascular pathology in dialysis patients and effective control over them seems to be an effective strategy aimed at increasing the duration and quality of life in patients receiving renal replacement therapy. The aim of the investigation was to study the species composition of colon microbiocenosis in patients with CKD receiving programmed HD treatment and to evaluate the effectiveness of its correction using a new immobilized synbiotic. Materials and methods: Samples of colon microbiota from 62 patients undergoing programmed hemodialysis were studied before and after a course of diet therapy that included probiotic components, in particular, the immobilized synbiotic LB-complex L. Isolation of microorganisms was carried out according to our original method; for bacteria identification, a MALDI-TOF Autoflex speed mass spectrometer (Bruker Daltonik, Germany) was used in the Biotyper program mode. The results were assessed using the criteria proposed by the authors and based on the OST 91500.11.0004-2003. The efficacy of the immobilized synbiotic was determined based on the clinical data, questionnaires, and bacteriological tests. Results: In patients receiving programmed hemodialysis (before the start of the diet therapy), chronic moderate inflammation and azotemia were found. Dysbiotic changes in microbiocenosis were revealed in all the examined patients; in the absence or suppression of lacto- and bifidoflora, the number and diversity of *Bacteroides* spp., *Clostridium* spp., *Collinsella* spp., *Eggerthella* spp. and other bacteria increased, which was consistent with the theory of functional redundancy of gut microbiota. From the answers to the questionnaires, a decrease in the quality of life was found (up to 70 points out of 100) according to six of the eight scales used. After the combined therapy using the synbiotic LB-complex L in the study group, 56% of the examined patients showed their microbiocenosis restored to normal; no grade III dysbiosis was detected in any patient. There was a significant decrease in CRP and ESR in these patients and an improvement in the quality of life by criteria reflecting physical health. Conclusion: Acute/chronic CVD in patients with CKD of the pre-dialysis and dialysis periods are the most frequent and formidable complications. The spectrum of "traditional" and "specific" CV risk factors in dialysis patients will be described in the chapter. Special attention will be paid to the intestinal microbiota and opportunistic intestinal microorganisms. *The aim* was to study the species composition of colon microbiocenosis in HD patients, and to evaluate the effectiveness of its correction using a new immobilized synbiotic. *Materials and Methods*. Samples of colon microbiota from 62 HD patients were studied before/after a course of diet therapy that included probiotic components, the immobilized synbiotic LB-complex L. MALDI-TOF Autoflex speed mass spectrometer was used in the Biotyper program mode. The efficacy of the immobilized synbiotic was determined based on the clinical data, questionnaires, and bacteriological tests. *Results*. Dysbiotic changes in microbiocenosis were revealed in all patients; in the absence/suppression of lacto-and bifidoflora, the number and diversity of *Bacteroides spp., Clostridium spp., Collinsella spp., Eggerthella spp.* and other bacteria increased. After the combined therapy using the synbiotic LB-complex L in the study group, 56% of the examined patients showed their microbiocenosis restored to normal; no grade III dysbiosis was detected in any patient.

Keywords: cerebrovascular disorders, specific risk factors, dialysis factors, calcification of the arterial microvasculature, anemia, uremic toxins, intestinal bacterial toxins, microbiocenosis, colon microbiota, chronic kidney disease, programmed hemodialysis, probiotics, synbiotics

1. Introduction

The prevalence of chronic kidney disease (CKD) is comparable to such socially significant diseases as hypertension, coronary artery disease, diabetes mellitus, obesity, metabolic syndrome throughout the world. The incidence is according to various sources 10–20% [1, 2]. The number of patients with CKD is progressively increasing and reaching the nature of a pandemic according to the opinion of some scientists [3, 4]. As a result, the number of patients receiving renal replacement therapy is growing (currently, more than 2 million people all over the world). In this connection, the share of the annual increase of dialysis programs is estimated at 6–12% [5].

1.1 Cerebrovascular disorders in patients undergoing long-term programmed hemodialysis (HD)

Cerebrovascular disorders in patients with CKD of the pre-dialysis and dialysis periods are usually classified as acute (transient ischemic attacks, ischemic and hemorrhagic strokes, subarachnoid hemorrhages) and chronic cerebrovascular diseases (chronic cerebral ischemia due to various variants of vascular cerebral microangiopathy (CMA), including cerebral amyloid angiopathy (CAA) and/or calcifying uremic arteriolopathy).

The remodeling of the micro- and macrocirculatory cerebral vessels continues in patients with dialysis stage of CKD, new vascular risk factors directly related to the dialysis procedure are aggravated and added, and cerebrovascular disorders progress [6]. It has been established that CKD and dialysis are also the causes of the development of CMA, which underlies the development of vascular cognitive impairments and acute cerebrovascular pathology. CMA is characterized by the damaged cerebral microvasculature (perforating cerebral arterioles, capillaries and venules) and damage of the white matter and brain nuclei [7–9]. In our studies, neuroimaging signs of CMA of varying severity were found in 100% of the examined patients who had been receiving renal replacement therapy with the long-term programmed HD. Expansion of perivascular spaces (100%) and white matter hyperintensity (81.4%) prevailed in the structure of MR signs of CMA. Cortical atrophy (67%), cerebral microbleeds (47%), asymptomatic lacunas (35.7%) and small subcortical infarctions (2.9%) were somewhat less common.

In dialysis patients, the risk of stroke and chronic cerebrovascular accidents increases multiple times, the risk of developing cognitive impairment is aggravated, and the quality of life of dialysis patients decreases [10, 11]. According to a meta-analysis conducted by Etgen in 2012, CKD is a statistically significant independent somatic risk factor for the development of cognitive impairment [12]. Epidemiological studies have also revealed a clear relationship between a decrease in glomerular filtration rate and high cardiovascular mortality in dialysis patients [13, 14], the proportion of which is extremely high among patients on renal replacement therapy [15]. According to our data, in patients undergoing programmed HD for more than 1-year, cognitive impairments were found much more often (75.5–81.1% of cases, $p = 0.05$) compared with people without renal pathology. The presence of ESRD and the presence of a patient on programmed HD, regardless of gender and educational level, can directly affect the development of cognitive impairment. For the screening assessment of the neuropsychological status of dialysis patients, the timely use of various neuropsychological scales is necessary: in particular, the use of the SLUMS and MoCA scales is possible. The risk factors for the development of cognitive impairment in persons receiving programmed HD can be considered an increase in the dialysis experience and the age of patients, as well as a low calculated dialysis adequacy index for urea (Kt/V less than 1.4).

In general, the problem of acute and chronic cerebrovascular disorders in dialysis patients remains the most urgent. Description of the spectrum of risk factors for cerebrovascular pathology in dialysis patients and effective control over them seems to be an effective strategy aimed at increasing the duration and quality of life in patients receiving renal replacement therapy.

1.2 Specific risk factors for the development of cerebrovascular pathology in patients with chronic kidney disease

Risk factors for cerebrovascular diseases in CKD and dialysis patients can be conditionally divided into "traditional" (arterial hypertension, diabetes mellitus, hypercholesterolemia) and "specific" (associated with renal pathology and dialysis procedures). Specific risk factors remain poorly understood and less well known to medical practitioners. The spectrum of specific factors of cerebrovascular risk in patients with dialysis stage of the CKD includes specific dialysis factors that form during programmed HD, as well as impaired phosphorus-calcium metabolism, increased blood levels of β2-microglobulin, homocysteine, malondialdehyde and superoxide dismutase, a decrease in the level of nitric oxide (II) metabolites, accumulation of uremic toxins and toxins of intestinal bacteria, development of nephrogenic anemia, dietary features of patients with renal pathology, etc.) [16–18]. Some of them are presented in more detail below.

1. Specific cerebrovascular risk factors that form during the HD procedure (dialysis factors) include disruptions of autoregulation of microcirculatory cerebral blood flow during regular programmed HD procedures, impaired drainage function of the brain against the background of stasis of interstitial fluid, aggravated by osmotic and electrolyte disorders of dialysis functioning of the glymphatic system. The high probability of developing hemodynamic instability and disruption of autoregulation of microcirculatory cerebral blood flow in dialysis patients, in addition to the traditional mechanisms common to patients with cardiovascular risk, may be due to the possibility of several specific complications during the HD procedure itself. In particular, during the programmed HD procedure, several patients may develop intradialysis hypotension, which is formed due to various pathogenetic mechanisms: the effect of ultrafiltration, hypovolemia and a decrease in the volume of extracellular fluid, an increase in body weight in the interdialysis period, electrolyte and osmolar disorders, and frequent autonomic dysfunction of dialysis patients. Also, in patients receiving programmed HD, intradialysis hypertension may develop due to an overestimation of the patient's "dry weight", intradialysis potassium drop, fluctuations in calcium levels, as well as the use of beta-blockers and other specific factors during the programmed HD procedure.

2. Violation of phosphorus-calcium metabolism and calcification of the arterial microvasculature: Already in the early stages of the development of CKD, there is a progressive impairment of phosphorus-calcium metabolism, which reaches its maximum during the dialysis period of CKD. These disorders include an excess of factors that contribute to the calcification of the arterial microvasculature, as well as a lack of factors that inhibit the calcification of the arterial wall. In the pathological circle of disorders of phosphorus-calcium metabolism and calcification of the arterial wall, several stages are distinguished. At the first stage, due to the presence of renal pathology and the development of CKD, there is a decrease in the excretion of phosphates in the urine and the formation of hyperphosphatemia. In response to an increase in serum phosphorus concentration, intestinal absorption of phosphorus decreases (it is discussed that this process is mediated by an increase in the level of phosphatonin (FGF23, fibroblast growth factor-23).

Long-term elevated levels of FGF23 in combination with destruction of the proximal renal tubules in CKD lead to a decrease in calcitriol levels, which means a decrease in calcium absorption in the intestine and suppression of its reabsorption in the kidneys, followed by the formation of hypocalcemia. At the next stage of the vicious circle of disorders of phosphorus-calcium metabolism, the loss of calcium by the body is compensated mainly due to the development of secondary hyperparathyroidism and increased resorption of bone tissue. When calcium is released from the bone, the level of serum phosphorus increases compensatory, thus, the vicious circle of phosphorus-calcium metabolism is closed [19]. Excess serum calcium is subsequently deposited in ectopic soft tissues and in the in the vascular system (in other words, vascular calcification is observed) [20]. It is believed that the process of calcification and increased stiffness of the vascular wall are associated with an increased risk of cardiovascular events, but there is no separate data on the cerebrovascular risk associated with arterial calcification and calcifying uremic arteriolopathy development [21]. The literature provides data on another possible mechanism by which an excess of phosphates leads to calcification of arteries, namely, a change in the phenotype of vascular smooth muscle cells (SMC) according to the "osteogenic type". Vascular wall SMCs stop producing SM22α-actin and instead synthesize bone formation factors involved in vascular calcification (alkaline phosphatase, osteocalcin) [22]. There is evidence that the mineralization of the vascular wall is also aggravated by the degradation of elastin against the background of the occurrence of osteogenically modified SMCs [23]. The degraded elastin increases the affinity of calcium and promotes the growth of hydroxyapatites along the elastic fibers. The gradual reduction of vascular smooth muscle leads to additional fibrosis of the median membrane of small and medium arteries, a decrease in cerebral blood flow and possible cerebrovascular risks. It is known that in CKD in the pre-dialysis period, there is also a lack of endogenous factors that inhibit the calcification of the arterial wall: FGF-23 klotho coreceptor, MGP protein (matrix glutamate protein), pyrophosphate, etc. reabsorption in the renal tubules [24]. The role of klotho as a protective factor of the vascular wall, which prevents osteogenic differentiation of SMCs, is discussed [25]. It is believed that as CKD progresses, the level of klotho gradually decreases, however, there is insufficient data on the effect of reduced concentrations of klotho on the development of cerebrovascular diseases [26]. Pyrophosphate and MGP protein (vitamin K-dependent glutamate-containing protein) are normally synthesized by healthy SMCs and inhibit vascular mineralization [27].

3. Anemia and dysfunction of blood cells: It is necessary to note another important specific risk factor for the development of cerebral vascular disorders in patients with CKD—the presence of anemia and dysfunction of blood cells, mainly platelets. The development of anemia in patients with CKD is associated with prolonged proteinuria, which is accompanied by losses of erythropoietin, transferrin and ionized iron, leading to a persistent decrease in hemoglobin levels [28]. As renal failure progresses, the anatomical structures that produce erythropoietin are gradually replaced by fibrous tissue, which is accompanied by the loss of hormone-producing properties. Observations by Chang et al. (2013), show that the presence of anemia in CKD increases the prevalence and severity of cerebrovascular disorders in patients with CKD [29]. The results of epidemiological studies indicate that the likelihood of developing an ischemic stroke is significantly higher in patients with anemia associated with CKD, and when the target values of hemoglobin and erythrocytes are reached, the risk of stroke is significantly reduced [30]. Platelet dysfunction in CKD is the result of a combination of intrinsic platelet abnormalities and disorders of platelet–vascular wall interaction [31]. This leads to a deterioration in platelet aggregation and impaired binding between the surface glycoprotein complex GPIIb/IIIa and fibrinogen on the subendothelial surface, thereby contributing to hypoaggregation and possible hemorrhagic events. The anemia that accompanies CKD exacerbates platelet dysfunction. This is due to a deficiency of erythropoietin, which normally improves platelet function by increasing the density of surface GPIIb/IIIa receptors [32]. There are works in the literature on the role of the transmembrane receptor RAGE in the formation of chronic vascular inflammation by inducing proinflammatory cytokines and chemokines. An increase in the concentration of end products of glycation observed in CKD patients due to impaired excretory function leads to an increase in the expression of RAGE in the cells of the vascular wall. This leads

to an increase in the concentration of sRAGE, the serum form of this receptor, which is a marker of inflammation and, in contrast to RAGE itself, can neutralize some of the inflammatory effects through competitive binding to circulating ligands [33]. In patients with CKD, the sRAGE level is 2.4 times higher than in the general population, and the concentration of proinflammatory ligands is 4 times higher than in the control group without CKD [34]. It is assumed that this may affect the formation of microangiopathy in the deep regions of the brain by activating the inflammatory response, impaired permeability of the blood–brain barrier and the occurrence of microbleeds [35], however, there is no convincing data on this yet.

4. Hyperhomocysteinemia and hyperβ2-microglobulinemia: Another specific risk factor for cerebrovascular disorders in CKD is hyperhomocysteinemia, which plays an important role in the formation of malignant atherosclerosis in CKD and thrombovascular disorders. Pathological accumulation of homocysteine occurs due to impaired reabsorption and metabolism of renal tubular cells in CKD [36]. β2-microglobulin is normally eliminated by the kidneys. Impaired elimination of β2-microglobulin from the body by the natural nephrogenic way leads to further deposition of amyloid in the walls of the microvasculature, the formation of secondary amyloidosis and CAA with the risk of cerebral microbleeds [17]. The high incidence of cerebral microbleeds (according to our data, 47% of the examined patients, mainly in the subcortical nuclei and supratentorial localization), can be explained by the development in this category of patients of both sporadic non-amyloid CMA and CAA, including against the background of persistent β2-microglobulinemia.

5. Accumulation of uremic toxins as a specific risk factor for cerebrovascular diseases in the pre-dialysis and dialysis periods of CKD. Uremic toxins can have both direct neurotoxic and vascular effects, and indirect, mediated through the aggravation of the negative effects of the above-described specific risk factors. It has been proven that the influence of such uremic toxins as uric acid, guanidine compounds, indoxyl sulfate, as well as proinflammatory cytokines–interleukins (Il) 1β, Il-6, tumor necrosis factor α, negatively affect cognitive functions and the functioning of the central nervous system under conditions of uremia [37]. The neurotoxic effects of these compounds can be mediated through ligand- and voltage-dependent calcium channels. Other studies have noted a direct effect of uremic toxins on the rate of cerebral blood flow [38]. It is believed that uremic toxins can enhance oxidative stress, chronic inflammation, endothelial dysfunction, and vascular calcification [39]. Studies in mice with CKD have shown that an increase in the level of a number of uremic toxins increases the content of intercellular adhesion molecules: VCAM-1 (CD106) and ICAM-1 (CD31) [40]. Cell adhesion molecules perform important functions of recognition, adhesion, and migration of immune-competent cells. In cases of violations of adhesive function of the endothelium and balance in the ratio of intercellular adhesion molecules, according to several authors, progression of angiopathy and malignant atherosclerosis is possible. In particular, it was found that uremic toxins induce the formation of angiopathy in patients with CKD, provoke calcification of the SMC of the aorta [41]. It is not yet known to what extent these mechanisms affect the development of cerebrovascular diseases, which requires further study of this issue.

6. Intestinal bacterial toxins: Another specific risk factor for the development of cerebral vascular disorders in patients with CKD, which will be presented

below in the form of an original study—intestinal bacterial toxins is distinguished. One of the negative consequences of the use of extracorporeal detoxification methods can be a violation of intestinal microbiocenosis. Recent studies have shown the presence of changes in intestinal microbiocenosis in patients with end-stage CKD. At the same time, in comparison with the predialysis stage patients, the patients receiving programmed HD had more pronounced disorders in the composition of the intestinal microbiota [42, 43]. At present time, the greatest attention is paid to two possible mechanisms for the development of changes in the composition of the intestinal microbiota in the literature: the characteristics of the diet and drugs taken in dialysis patients, as well as the regimen of the selected method of extracorporeal detoxification (HD, PD, or a functioning kidney transplant). Opportunistic gut microorganisms can produce uremic toxins, in particular, indoxyl sulfate and paracresol sulfate, which are associated with an increased risk of inflammation, increased oxidative stress, progression of CKD, and a higher risk of cardiovascular disease (CVD), which appears to predispose to disorders of intestinal microbiocenosis and mediated vascular risks.

Restrictions on the consumption of fruits and vegetables (sources of potassium), cheese, milk and dairy products (sources of phosphorus) contribute to the predominance of bacteria that produce toxic metabolites [44], which negatively affects the integrity of colonocytes and impairs the protective barrier of the colon mucosa [45]. Insufficient protein intake and loss of albumin during dialysis, especially when using high-flux membranes, also lead to a change in the species structure of the intestinal microbiome and increase the risk of bacterial translocation (penetration of microorganisms from the lumen of the gastrointestinal tract through the mucous barrier into the blood and lymph flow) and endotoxemia [42, 46]. On the contrary, if a high-fiber diet is properly followed in patients on PD, circulating concentrations of uremic toxins (in particular, paracresol sulfate) and some other markers of inflammation are reduced [47–49]. The dialysis procedure itself is associated with inevitable dietary restrictions for the dialysis patient, which may partly explain the differences between patients on PH and PD [50]. Thus, patients receiving PD are less prone to hyperkalemia than patients receiving PD [51]. Dietary restrictions in this category of patients are considered milder, and the diet is more varied.

Patients receiving renal replacement therapy are forced to take several medications regularly, which, as well as dietary habits, can negatively affect the composition of the intestinal microbiocenosis. However, the data on this issue are inconsistent. In particular, Khoury et al. (2016), postulate that the frequent use of antibiotics and phosphate binders in patients with end-stage CKD can alter the composition of the intestinal microbiota and, therefore, jeopardize the intestinal barrier [52]. Researchers consider phosphate binders, immunosuppressants, antibiotics, and proton pump inhibitors as drugs that negatively affect the intestinal microbiocenosis of dialysis patients [53].

The aim of our investigation was to study the species composition of colon microbiocenosis in patients with CKD receiving programmed HD treatment and to evaluate the effectiveness of its correction using a new immobilized synbiotic.

2. Materials and methods

The examined patients were on planned outpatient treatment in the department of gravitational surgery of blood and hemodialysis in 2018–2020. Patients were enrolled in this parallel-group randomized controlled clinical trial using a continuous sample method. The study involved 62 patients, including 36 women (58.1%) and 26 men (41.9%). Inclusion criteria were: age from 18 to 85 years; the presence of the dialysis stage of chronic kidney disease, the experience of program hemodialysis for more than 1 year; the adequacy of the programmed hemodialysis (at least 3 sessions per week, at least 4 hours/session and 720 minutes per week, the calculated dialysis adequacy index (purification coefficient Kt/V for urea) is at least 1.4, calculated based on the proportion of urea reduction weight loss during dialysis, dialysis time and patient weight); no antibiotic intake for 2 months and more, signed informed consent of the patient.

The patients were divided into the main group and the comparison group matched by sex and age. Basic therapy for patients with dialysis stage CKD of both groups included a high-protein diet and, if necessary, the appointment of drug therapy: antihypertensive—β-blockers (bisoprolol), blockers of Ca-channel (amlodipine), blockers of imidazoline receptors (moxonidine) and hypolipidemic—atorvastatin or rosuvastatin; as well as the treatment of anemia: erythropoietin α (or β) or methoxypolyethylene-glycol-epoetin-β; iron preparations (iron (III) hydroxide sucrose complex); correction of mineral-bone disorders: active metabolites of vitamin D (calcitriol, paricalcitol), calcimimetics (cinacalcet), phosphate-binding agents (β-iron (III) oxyhydroxide complex); correction of protein-energy deficiency (keto analogs of amino acids) [43].

The main group consisted of 32 patients with dialysis stage of CKD, including 19 women (59%) and 13 men (41%) aged 38–65 years (mean age 57.1 ± 7.9 years). Dialysis experience—from 12 to 123 months (40.6 ± 29.8 months). They received basic therapy and, as a probiotic, a new immobilized synbiotic "LB-complex L". The comparison group included 30 patients, including 17 women (57%) and 13 men (43%) aged 34–65 years (54.7 ± 8.4 years) with comparable dialysis experience. They received basic therapy and a placebo. All patients underwent an assessment of the nature of complaints, clinical and laboratory data (general blood test with determination of the number of leukocytes, ESR; biochemical blood test with determination of creatinine, blood urea, C-reactive protein); the dialysis adequacy index (purification coefficient Kt/V for urea) was calculated for each patient. The quality of life was assessed using the SF-36 (Short form medical outcomes study) questionnaire [11]. The study of the species composition of the intestinal microbiota and the assessment of the state of the microbiocenosis was carried out using the unified methodology developed by us and OST 91500.11.0004-2003 "Patient Management Protocol. Intestinal dysbiosis" [54, 55]. Microorganisms were identified on an autoflex speed time-of-flight MALDI-TOF mass spectrometer (Bruker Daltonik, Germany) using the Biotyper 4.1.80 RTC program. The author's immobilized multistrain synbiotic LB-complex L (SGR RU.77.99.88.003.E.002522.06.18) [56], recommended as a source of probiotic microorganisms (bifidobacteria and lactobacilli) and zeolites (enterosorbent), which increase the body's nonspecific resistance and have a detoxifying effect. Six strains that make up the synbiotic under study belong to species with a documented history of safe use and are approved for the production of medical immunobiological preparations. They do not have genetically modified analogues, meet the requirements for probiotic strains [36, 57], in particular, they have high antagonistic activity against a wide range of pathogenic and opportunistic microorganisms, antibiotic resistance undetermined by plasmids, and are sufficiently resistant to the action of gastric juice and bile. Zeolites of the Kholinsky deposit, selected as a matrix for the immobilization of probiotic strains, are approved for use in medical practice (SGR KZ.16.01.78.003.E.004706.08.15 from 18.08.2015). A unique property of clinoptilolites is the property of selective ion exchange: they are ultra-elements, if they are not enough, and they remove substances that are in excess from the body. Zeolites have pronounced sorption properties, since the openwork of the crystal lattice creates a large adsorption volume, they do not break down and do not undergo any changes in the human body [19]. Statistical processing was performed using standard software packages Statistica 6.1 and Microsoft Excel 2007. Data were presented as arithmetic mean (M) and standard error of the mean (m). If the distribution of data in the samples was not characterized as normal, nonparametric methods of analysis were used. The significance of the differences was assessed using the Mann–Whitney test. Differences between independent groups were considered statistically significant with a probability of error $p < 0.05$.

3. Results and discussion

At the beginning of this study, a comprehensive examination of patients on programmed HD was carried out, including the determination of clinical and laboratory parameters, an assessment of the quality of life by a questionnaire method and a bacteriological analysis of the colon microbiocenosis.

When analyzing laboratory data before using the synbiotic, comparable indicators were found in both groups: a moderate increase in ESR (43.7 ± 21.4 and 42.4 ± 18.9 mm/h) and CRP (6.8 ± 3.1 and 6.5 ± 2.9 g/L), normal leukocyte count (6.7–6.8*10^9/L), increased levels of blood urea (19.6–19.4 mmol/L) and blood creatinine (697.1–688.5 μmol/L), indicating the presence of chronic moderate inflammation and azotemia in patients receiving PG. The Kt/V index for urea was 1.43 ± 0.16 and 1.41 ± 0.18, which indicated the adequacy of the dialysis dose (**Table 1**).

ESR, erythrocyte sedimentation rate; C-RP, C-reactive protein; Le, leukocyte count; Kt/V for urea index, the dialysis adequacy index (for urea).

An in-depth study of the microbiota in patients with CKD undergoing hemodialysis showed that among representatives of the phylum Actinobacteria in the microbiocenosis of the colon, representatives of the genus *Bifidobacterium* are found in 75% of the examined, in 43.7% of them the detected number of bifidobacteria is significantly lower than normal. 1–2 species of bifidobacteria were isolated from each patient, and *Bifidobacterium longum* prevailed in the species structure −43.75% (**Figures 1–4**).

Using our technique, in this study, such rarely identified species of the Enterobacteriaceae family as *Enterobacter asburiae*, *Enterobacter kobei*, *Citrobacter youngae*, *Serratia liquefaciens*, and *Raoultella planticola* were isolated.

Dysbiotic changes in colon microbiocenosis of varying degrees were detected in 100% of the examined patients (**Figure 5**).

During the analysis of the composition of the intestinal microbiota, it was noted that in the absence or suppression of lacto- and bifidoflora, the number and species diversity of microorganisms of the genera *Bacteroides*, *Clostridium*, *Collinsella*, *Eggerthella*, etc. literature [58]. The concept of functional redundancy has been validated in metagenomic studies. For example, in experimental models

	ESR, mm/hour	C-RP, g/L	Le, cell/L	Urea (blood), mMol/L	Creatinine (blood), μmol/L	Kt/V for urea index
Study group	43.7 ± 21.4	6.8 ± 3.1	6.7·10^9/L	19.6	697.1	1.43 ± 0.16
Control group	42.4 ± 18.9	6.5 ± 2.9	6.8·10^9/L	19.4	688.5	1.41 ± 0.18

Table 1.
Values of some clinical laboratory test hematology and blood chemistry indicators in study and control groups.

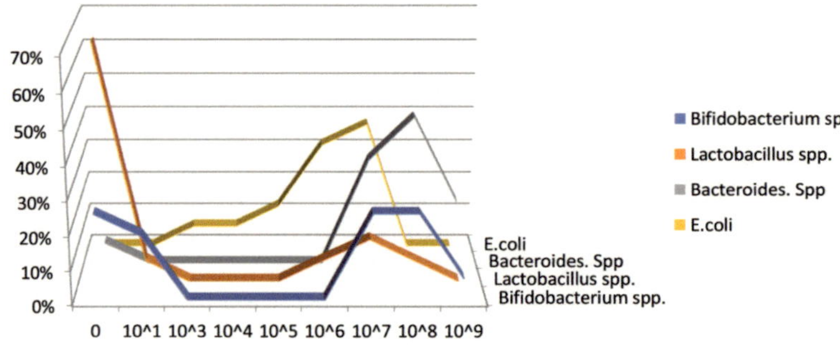

Figure 1.
Quantitative characteristics of major components of the obligate intestinal microbiota in patients with chronic kidney disease receiving programmed hemodialysis.

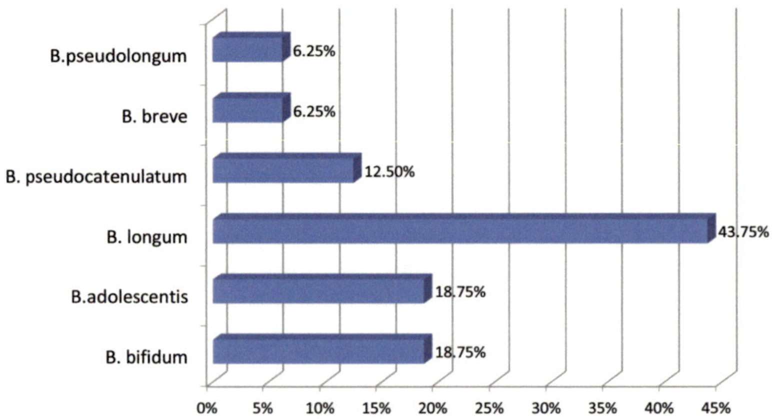

Figure 2.
Occurrence rates for various species of the genus Bifidobacterium in patients with chronic kidney disease receiving programmed hemodialysis.

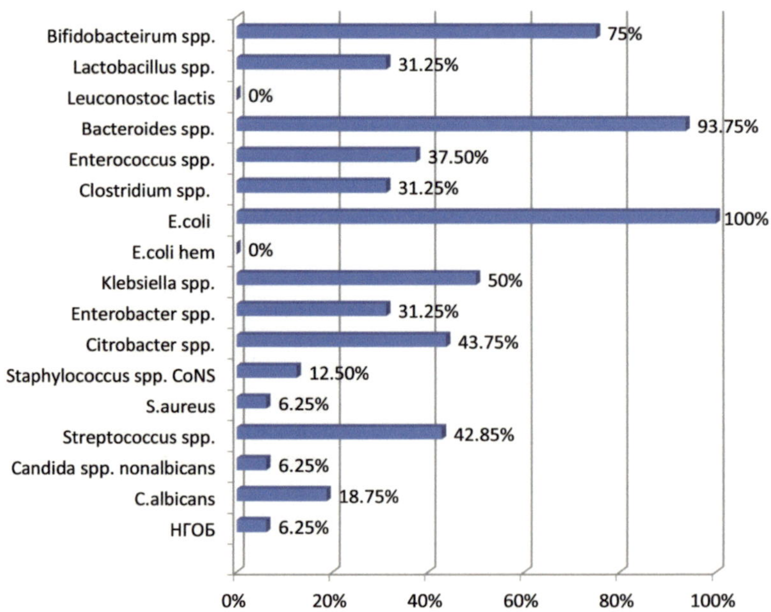

Figure 3.
Occurrence rates for various species of the normal human colon microbiota in patients with chronic kidney disease receiving programmed hemodialysis.

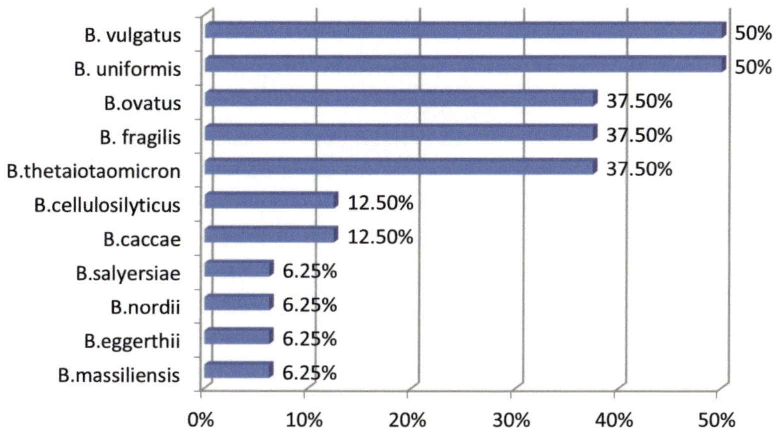

Figure 4.
Occurrence rates for various species of the genus Bacteroides spp. in patients with chronic kidney disease receiving programmed hemodialysis.

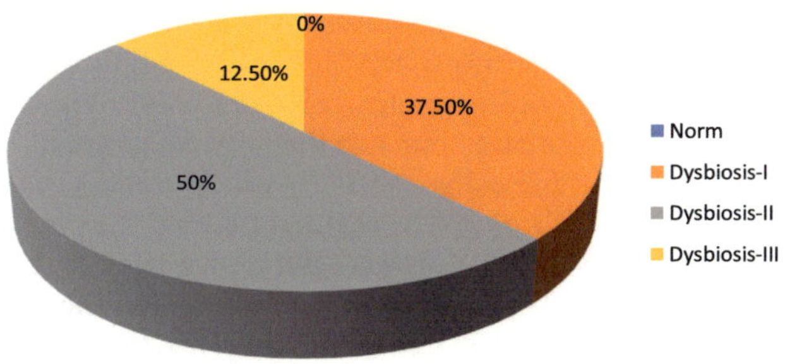

Figure 5.
Dysbiotic disorders (grades I–III) of the colon microbiocenosis in patients with chronic kidney disease receiving programmed hemodialysis before starting treatment with symbiotic.

[59], it was clearly shown how, on the one hand, functional redundancy and, on the other hand, metabolic "specialization" (production of lactate and acetate) of representatives of the two main bacterial phyla—Firmicutes and Bacteroides—provide stability the gut ecosystem as a whole. However, in CKD, due to the progression of renal failure, the concentration of uremic toxins in the intra- and extracellular spaces increases, which leads to their influx into the gastrointestinal tract. With the help of bacterial urease, urea is quickly converted into ammonium hydroxide, irritating of the mucous membrane of the large intestine and, in the future, the development of inflammation. Approximately 68% of creatinine is transformed by bacteria into creatine, and the remainder is converted into 1-methylhydantoin, sarcosine, methylguanidine, etc., by the quantitatively prevailing proteolytic microorganisms (*B. fragilis*, *Bacteroides thetaiotaomicron*, *Enterobacter* spp., *Citrobacter* spp.) recognized as uremic toxins, which contribute to the aggravation of the manifestations of renal failure [21, 60].

Thus, in pathological conditions in humans, the mechanism of functional redundancy of the microbiota can lead to a worsening of the course of the disease [20]. As a result, the restoration of microbiocenosis with the help of undoubtedly probiotic microorganisms (lactobacilli and bifidobacteria) is of particular importance: proteolytic bacteria are excluded from the pathogenesis of the underlying disease formate and succinate) remains unchanged.

After complex therapy, both in the control group and in the group in which the synbiotic "LB-complex L" was used [9], bifidobacteria were detected in 100% of cases.

However, in the main group, they were isolated mainly in amounts of 109–1010 CFU/g, while in the comparison group, their number was 107–108 CFU/g ($p < 0.05$). Lactobacilli were isolated in amounts of 107–108 CFU/g in 100% of patients in the main group and 56.25% of those examined from the comparison group. In 43.75% of patients in the comparison group, lactobacilli were absent in the microbiocenosis. Bacteroids were detected in 100% of the examined in the amount of 108–109 CFU/g in the main group and 106–107 CFU/g in the comparison group ($p < 0.05$).

In the main group, opportunistic microorganisms after treatment were detected with a lower frequency and in a smaller amount than in the comparison group. Thus, *Klebsiella* spp. was isolated in 6.25% versus 50.0% in the comparison group, *Citrobacter* spp.—in 12.5 and 56.25%, respectively. A similar trend was observed about other opportunistic microorganisms and fungi (*Raoultella* spp., *Enterococcus* spp., *Streptococcus* spp., *Acinetobacter* spp., *Corynebacterium* spp., *Microbacterium* spp., *Bacillus* spp., *Candida* spp., etc.). Thus, in the main group, 56% of the examined microbiocenosis recovered, grade III dysbiosis was not detected in any patient. In the comparison group, the microbiological indicators worsened: the number of cases of detection of pronounced microbiocenosis disorders of II and III degrees increased. In clinical and biochemical blood parameters of patients of the main group, attention is drawn to the decrease after treatment in the level of inflammation indicators—CRP (5.3 g/L) and ESR (36.2 mm/h).

The modern concept of providing medical care requires not only the restoration of the biological function of the body but also the normalization of its functioning. When assessing the quality of life using the SF-36 questionnaire, our study revealed an improvement in these indicators on the scales reflecting the physical component of health in the main group. The most positive dynamics after the treatment in the main group was noted on such scales of quality of life as RP—the scale of role activity due to a physical condition (before treatment: 39.2, after: 45.1); P, pain intensity scale (65.2 and 71.3, respectively) and GH, general health scale (52.6 and 58.8, respectively) (**Figure 6**) [60].

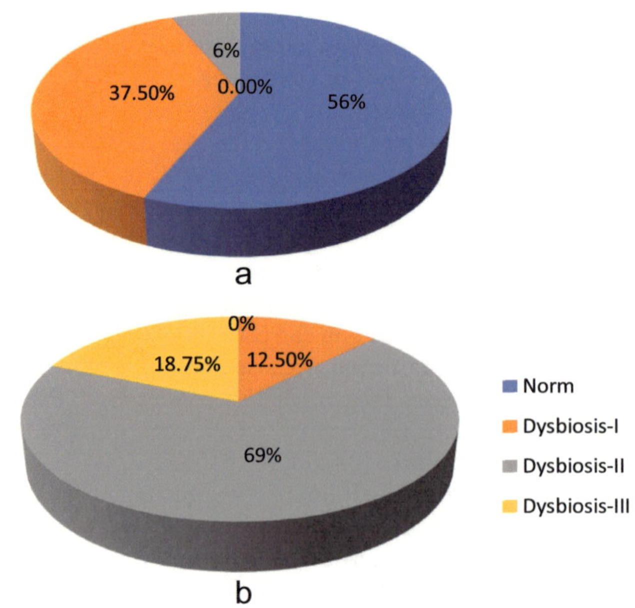

Figure 6.
Dysbiotic disorders of colon microbiocenosis in patients with chronic kidney disease receiving programmed hemodialysis after treatment (a) main group; (b) comparison group.

4. Conclusion

Thus, acute and chronic cerebrovascular disorders in patients with CKD of the pre-dialysis and dialysis periods are the most frequent and formidable complications that develop against the background of "traditional" and "specific" cerebrovascular risk factors. Because of the studies, new knowledge was obtained about the species diversity and species representation of the microbiocenosis of the colon lumen in patients with chronic kidney disease receiving program dialysis. The inclusion of the author's immobilized multistrain synbiotic "LB-complex L" as a dietary component in the basic therapy allows not only to restore the evolutionarily determined microbiocenosis, but also improves the quality of life of patients, and also helps to reduce the risk of cardiovascular events.

Active control of the described specific indicators (impaired phosphorus-calcium metabolism and calcification of the arterial bed, correction of anemia and dysfunction of blood corpuscles, hyperhomocysteinemia and hyperβ2-microglobulinemia, accumulation of uremic toxins and toxins of intestinal bacteria, correction of pathologically altered intestinal microbiocenosis) and conditions of dialysis their timely prevention, as well as the correction of intradialysis hypo-/hypertension, are necessary for the timely prevention of cerebrovascular disorders in dialysis patients.

Author details

Alexey E. Khrulev[1]*, Irina V. Belova[2], Irina V. Soloveva[2], Anna G. Tochilina[2], Natalya A. Shiyanova[1], Anastasiya A. Nikitina[1] and Natalya S. Khruleva[1]

1 Privolzhsky Research Medical University, Nizhny Novgorod, Russia

2 Academician I.N. Blokhina Nizhny Novgorod Scientific Research Institute of Epidemiology and Microbiology, Nizhny Novgorod, Russia

*Address all correspondence to: alexey_khrulev@mail.ru

References

[1] Couser WG, Remuzzi G, Mendis S, Tonelli M. The contribution of chronic kidney disease to the global burden of major noncommunicable diseases. Kidney International. 2011;**80**(12): 1258-1270. DOI: 10.1038/ki.2011.368

[2] Kidney Disease: Improving Global Outcomes (KDIGO) CKD Work Group. KDIGO 2012 clinical practice guideline for the evaluation and management of chronic kidney disease. Kidney International. Supplement. 2013;**3**:1-150

[3] Tomilina NA, Bikbov BT. Renal replacement therapy for end-stage renal disease patients in Russian Federation, 1998-2011 (Report of the Russian Registry of renal replacement therapy). Vestnik Transplantologii i Iskusstvennykh Organov. 2015;**17**(1):35-58. DOI: 10.15825/1995-1191-2015-1-35-58

[4] Vasilyeva IA. Life quality peculiarities among patients with chronic renal failure treated by hemodialysis. Izvestiya Rossiiskogo Gosudarstvennogo Pedagogicheskogo Universiteta Imeni A.I.Gertsena. 2008;**57**:75-86

[5] Shutov AM. Chronic kidney disease is a global problem of the XXI century. Klinicheskaya meditsina. 2014;**92**(5):5-10

[6] Kosovskikh AA, Churlyaev YA, Kan SL, Lyzlov AN, Kirsanov TV, Vartanyan AR. Central hemodynamics and microcirculation in critical conditions. General Reanimatology= Obshchaya Reanimatologiya. 2013;**9**(1):18. DOI: 10.15360/1813-9779-2013-1-18

[7] Wardlaw JM, Smith C, Dichgans M. Small vessel disease: Mechanisms and clinical implications. The Lancet Neurology. 2019;**18**(7):684-696. DOI: 10.1016/S1474-4422(19)30079-1

[8] Khrulev AE, Tolbuzova DD, Plokhenko EA, Egorova PA, Sorokoumova SN, Suvorova OV, et al. Cognitive status and risk factors for cognitive impairment in dialysis patients. General Reanimatology (Obshchaya Reanimatologiya). 2020;**16**(4):21-31. DOI: 10.15360/1813-9779-2020-4-21-31

[9] Tsai Y-H, Lee M, Lin L-C, Chang S-W, Weng H-H, Yang J-T, et al. Association of chronic kidney disease with small vessel disease in patients with hypertensive intracerebral hemorrhage. Frontiers in Neurology. 2018;**9**:284. DOI: 10.3389/fneur.2018.00284

[10] Khrulev AE, Studyanikova SF, Langraf SV, Sadyrin RV, Grigor'eva VN. Cognitive impairment in patients on hemodialysis. Neurology Bulletin= Nevrologicheskij vestnik. 2019;**51**(2): 36-40. DOI: 10.17816/nb15659

[11] Khrulev AE, Kudryavtseva ES, Egorova PA, Rodionova AD, Sorokoumova SN, Suvorova OV. Quality of life of long-term hemodialysis patients. General Reanimatology=Obshchaya Reanimatologiya. 2019;**15**(2):4-12. DOI: 10.15360/1813-9779-2019-2-4-12

[12] Etgen T, Chonchol M, Förstl H, Sander D. Chronic kidney disease and cognitive impairment: A systematic review and meta-analysis. American Journal of Nephrology. 2012;**35**(5): 474-482. DOI: 10.1159/000338135

[13] Go AS, Chertow GM, Fan D, et al. Chronic kidney disease and the risks of death, cardiovascularevents, and hospitalization. The New England Journal of Medicine. 2004;**351**(13):1296-1305. DOI: 10.1056/NEJMoa041031

[14] Tonelli M, Wiebe N, Culleton B, House A, Rabbat C, Fok M, et al. Chronic kidney disease and mortality risk: A systematic review. Journal of the American Society of Nephrology. 2006;**17**(7):2034-2047. DOI: 10.1681/ASN.2005101085

[15] Litovkina ON, Nekipelova EV, Sirotina SS, Efremova O, Sorokina IN. Polymorphism of vascular homeostasis genes and progression of chronic kidney disease in patients with chronic glomerulonephritis. Research Journal of Pharmaceutical, Biological and Chemical Sciences. 2014;**5**(5):1079-1082

[16] Guo H, Liu W, Li H, Yang J. Structural and functional brain changes in hemodialysis patients with end-stage renal disease: DTI analysis results and ALFF analysis results. International Journal of Nephrology and Renovascular Disease. 2021;**14**:77-86. DOI: 10.2147/IJNRD.S295025

[17] Khrulev AE, Nikitina AA, Khruleva NS. Specific risk factors for cerebrovascular disorders in patients with chronic kidney disease in the pre-dialysis period. Cardiovascular Therapy and Prevention (Kardiovaskulyarnaya terapiya i profilaktika). 2019;**18**(3):88-93. DOI: 10.15829/1728-8800-2019-3-88-93

[18] Khrulev AE, Solovyeva IV, Khruleva NS, Grigoryeva VN, Belova IV, Tochilina AG, et al. Intestinal microbiota as a significant factor of endotoxemia and vascular risk in patients on hemodialysis. Practical Medicine. 2019;**17**(8):11-16

[19] Mineral and osteal disorders in chronic kidney disease (MOD-CKD). Available from: http://nonr.ru/wp-content/uploads/2013/11/Минеральные-и-костные-нарушения-прихронической-болезни-почек.pdf [Accessed: 08 May 2018]

[20] Hruska K, Mathew S, Lund R, et al. Hyperphosphatemia of chronic kidney disease. Kidney International. 2008; **4**(2):148-157. DOI: 10.1038/ki.2008.130

[21] Lau WL, Ix JH. Clinical detection, risk factors, and cardiovascular consequences of medial arterial calcification: A pattern of vascular injury associated with aberrant mineral metabolism. Seminars in Nephrology. 2013;**33**(2):93-105. DOI: 10.1016/j.semnephrol.2012.12.011

[22] Steitz SA, Speer MY, Curinga G, et al. Smooth muscle cell phenotypic transition associated with calcification: Upregulation of Cbfa1 and down-regulation of smooth muscle lineage markers. Circulation Research. 2001; **89**(12):1147-1154. DOI: 10.1161/hh2401.101070

[23] Hosaka N, Mizobuchi M, Ogata H, et al. Elastin degradation accelerates phosphate induced mineralization of vascular smooth muscle cells. Calcified Tissue International. 2009;**85**(6):523-529

[24] Gattineni J, Bates C, Twombley K, et al. FGF23 decreases renal NaPi-2a and NaPi-2c expression and induces hypophosphatemia in vivo predominantly via FGF receptor 1. American Journal of Physiology. Renal Physiology. 2009;**297**(2):282-291. DOI: 10.1152/ajprenal.90742.2008

[25] Chen T, Mao H, Chen C, et al. The role and mechanism of α-Klotho in the calcification of rat aortic vascular smooth muscle cells. BioMed Research International. 2015;**2015**:1-7. DOI: 10.1155/2015/194362

[26] Hu MC, Shi M, Zhang J, et al. Klotho deficiency causes vascular calcification in chronic kidney disease. Journal of the American Society of Nephrology. 2011;**22**(1):124-136. DOI: 10.1681/ASN.2009121311

[27] Schurgers LJ, Barreto DV, Barreto FC, et al. The circulating inactive form of matrix gla protein is a surrogate marker for vascular calcification in chronic kidney disease: A preliminary report. Clinical Journal of the American Society of Nephrology. 2010;**5**(4):568-575. DOI: 10.2215/CJN.07081009

[28] Korzh AN. Cadiorenal syndrome in patients with cronic kidney disease and

coronary heart disease. Pochki. 2015;**1**: 45-51

[29] Chang YL, Hung SH, Ling W, et al. Association between ischemic stroke and irondeficiency anemia: A population-based study. PLoS One. 2013;**8**(12):1-7. DOI: 10.1371/journal.pone.0082952

[30] Seliger SL, Zhang AD, Weir MR, et al. Erythropoiesis-stimulating agents increase the risk of acute stroke in patients with chronic kidney disease. Kidney International. 2011;**80**:288-294. DOI: 10.1038/ki.2011.49

[31] Chan KE, Lazarus JM, Thadhani R, et al. Anticoagulant and antiplatelet usage associates with mortality among hemodialysis patients. Journal of the American Society of Nephrology. 2009;**20**:872-881. DOI: 10.1681/ASN.2008080824

[32] Lau WL, Huisa BN, Fisher M. The cerebrovascular-chronic kidney disease connection: Perspectives and mechanisms. Translational Stroke Research. 2017;**8**:67-76

[33] Charidimou A, Werring DJ. A raging fire in acute lacunar stroke: Inflammation, bloodbrain barrier dysfunction and the origin of cerebral. Journal of the Neurological Sciences. 2014;**340**(1-2):1-2. DOI: 10.1016/j.jns.2014.03.004

[34] Xiao L, Sun W, Lan W, et al. Correlation between cerebral microbleeds and S100B/RAGE in acute lacunar stroke patients. Journal of the Neurological Sciences. 2014;**340**(1-2):208-212. DOI: 10.1016/j.jns.2014.03.006

[35] Isoyama N, Leurs P, Qureshi AR, et al. Plasma S100A12 and soluble receptor of advanced glycation end product levels and mortality in chronic kidney disease stage 5 patients. Nephrology, Dialysis, Transplantation. 2015;**30**(1):84-91. DOI: 10.1093/ndt/gfu259

[36] Nesterenko OV, Borodulin VB, Goremykin VI, et al. Importance of hyperhomocysteinemia (HHC) in chronic pyelonephritis. Fundamental Research. 2014;**7**(1):193-196

[37] Watanabe K, Watanabe T, Nakayama M. Cerebro-renal interactions: Impact of uremic toxins on cognitive function. Neurotoxicology. 2014;**44**:184-193. DOI: 10.1016/j.neuro.2014.06.014

[38] Bugnicourt JM, Da Silveira C, Bengrine A, et al. Chronic renal failure alters endothelial function in cerebral circulation in mice. American Journal of Physiology. Heart and Circulatory Physiology. 2011;**301**:1143-1152. DOI: 10.1152/ajpheart.01237.2010

[39] Watanabe H, Miyamoto Y, Otagiri M, et al. Update on the pharmacokinetics and redox properties of protein-bound uremic toxins. Journal of Pharmaceutical Sciences. 2011;**100**:3682-3695. DOI: 10.1002/jps.22592

[40] Six I, Maizel J, Barreto FC, et al. Effects of phosphate on vascular function under normal conditions and influence of the uraemic state. Cardiovascular Research. 2012;**96**: 130-139. DOI: 10.1093/cvr/cvs240

[41] Muteliefu G, Enomoto A, Jiang P, et al. Indoxyl sulphate induces oxidative stress and the expression of osteoblast-specific proteins in vascular smooth muscle cells. Nephrology, Dialysis, Transplantation. 2009;**24**:2051-2058. DOI: 10.1093/ndt/gfn757

[42] Nistor I, Palmer SC, Craig JC, et al. Haemodiafiltration, haemofiltration and haemodialysis for end-stage kidney disease. Cochrane Database of Systematic Reviews. 2015;**5**:CD006258

[43] Andrusev AM, Bevzenko AY, Vishnevskiy KA, Gerasimchuk RP, Zemchenkov AY, Nazarov AV, et al. Recommendations of the Russian Dialysis Society for assessing the quality of medical care in preparation for the initiation of renal replacement therapy

and dialysis treatment for adult patients with stage V CKD. Nefrologia i dializ. 2015;**17**(1):10-19

[44] Lau WL, Kalantar-Zadeh K, Vaziri ND. The gut as a source of inflammation in chronic kidney disease. Nephron. 2015;**130**:92-98

[45] Vaziri ND, Zhao YY, Pahl MV. Altered intestinal microbial flora and impaired epithelial barrier structure and function in CKD: The nature, mechanisms, consequences and potential treatment. Nephrology, Dialysis, Transplantation. 2016;**31**:737-746

[46] Webster A, Nistor I. Haemodiafiltration, haemofiltration and haemodialysis for end-stage kidney disease. Nephrology. 2016;**21**(6):526-527

[47] Sirich TL, Plummer NS, Gardner CD, et al. Effect of increasing dietary fiber on plasma levels of colon-derived solutes in hemodialysis patients. Clinical Journal of the American Society of Nephrology. 2014;**9**:1603-1610

[48] Shi K, Wang F, Jiang H, et al. Gut bacterial translocation may aggravate microinflammation in hemodialysis patients. Digestive Diseases and Sciences. 2014;**59**(9):2109-2117

[49] Xie LM, Ge YY, Huang X, et al. Effects of fermentable dietary fiber supplementation on oxidative and inflammatory status in hemodialysis patients. International Journal of Clinical and Experimental Medicine. 2015;**8**(1):1363-1369

[50] Crespo-Salgado J. Intestinal microbiota in pediatric patients with end stage renal disease: A Midwest Pediatric Nephrology Consortium study. Microbiome. 2016;**4**:50

[51] Wang AY. ISPD cardiovascular and metabolic guidelines in adult peritoneal dialysis patients part I—Assessment and management of various cardiovascular risk factors. Peritoneal Dialysis International. 2015;**35**:379-387

[52] Khoury T, Tzukert K, Abel R, et al. The gut-kidney axis in chronic renal failure: A new potential target for therapy. Hemodialysis International. 2017;**21**:323-334

[53] Zhernakova A et al. Population-based metagenomics analysis reveals markers for gut microbiome composition and diversity. Science. 2016;**352**:565-569

[54] Tochilina AG, Belova IV, Solov'eva IV, Zhirnov VA, Ivanova TP. Criteria for evaluating the composition of the colon lumen biocenosis. Spravochnik zaveduyushchego KDL. 2016;**8**:54-78

[55] Otraslevoy standart OST 91500.11.0004-2003. Protokol vedeniya bol'nykh. Disbakterioz kishechnika: Prikaz MZ RF No.231 [Industry standard OST 91500.11.0004-2003. Patient management protocol. Intestinal dysbiosis: Order of the Ministry of Health of the Russian Federation No. 231]. Moscow; 2003; 112 p

[56] Belova IV, Tochilina AG, Soloveva IV, Zhilenkova OG, Melikhova AV, Belyaeva EV, et al. The results of "LB-complex L" immobilized synbiotic safety study in animals. Mezhdunarodnyy zhurnal prikladnykh i fundamental'nykh issledovaniy. 2018;**2**:85-89

[57] Kuzmichev DE, Skrebov RV, Chirkov SV, et al. Amyloidosis. Zdravoohranenie Ugry: opyt i innovacii. 2016;**1**:59-64

[58] Sitkin SI, Tkachenko EI, Vakhitov TY. Metabolic dysbiosis of the gut microbiota and its biomarkers. Eksperimental'naa i klinicheskaa gastroenterologia. 2015;**12**:6-29

[59] Mahowald MA, Rey FE, Seedorf H, Turnbaugh PJ, Fulton RS, Wollam A, et al. Characterizing a model human gut microbiota composed of members of its

two dominant bacterial phyla. Proceedings of the National Academy of Sciences of the United States of America. 2009;**106**(14):5859-5864. DOI: 10.1073/pnas.0901529106

[60] Belova IV, Khrulev AE, Tochilina AG, Khruleva NS, Lobanova NA, Zhirnov VA, et al. Colon microbiocenosis and its correction in patients receiving programmed hemodialysis. Sovremennye tehnologii v medicine. 2020;**12**(5):62-70. DOI: 10.17691/stm2020.12.5.07

Chapter 7

Enzyme-Replacement Therapy in Fabry Disease

Hanny Sawaf, Angelika L. Erwin, Fang Zhao, Tushar J. Vachharajani and Xiangling Wang

Abstract

Fabry disease is a rare X-linked lysosomal storage disorder due to mutations in the GLA gene causing complete or partial deficiency of the lysosomal enzyme alpha-galactosidase A (a-Gal A). This enzyme deficiency results in tissue accumulation of trihexosylceramide causing the diseases' systemic manifestations, including acroparesthesia, angiokeratomas, cardiac disease, cerebrovascular manifestations, and kidney disease. Kidney manifestations of Fabry disease can include proteinuria, renal tubular dysfunction, hypertension, and cystic formation. With the relatively recent introduction of enzyme-replacement therapy (ERT), this congenital disorder can now be treated providing these patients with much longer life expectancies and less severe systemic manifestations than before. When started in the appropriate population, ERT is generally continued until a reason for stopping therapy arises. Although ERT is expensive, it has drastically changed the clinical outcome of patients with Fabry disease, and timely initiation of ERT and regular assessments of disease progression by a multidisciplinary care team are critical for the long-term management of these patients.

Keywords: Fabry disease, GLA gene, alpha-galactosidase A, trihexosylceramide, enzyme-replacement therapy, glycosphingolipids, agalsidase, kidney disease, zebra bodies

1. Introduction

Fabry disease (OMIM # 301500), also called Anderson-Fabry disease, is a rare X-linked lysosomal storage disorder due to mutations in the *GLA* gene, causing complete or partial deficiency of the lysosomal enzyme alpha-galactosidase A (α-Gal A) [1, 2]. The incidence of Fabry disease is estimated at 1:50,000 to 1:117,000 in males [3]. It has been found among all demographic, ethnic, and racial groups. Fabry disease has been recognized as a heterogeneous, highly complex, and multi-systemic disease associated with a high burden of morbidity and mortality [2].

The α-Gal A enzyme is crucial for glycosphingolipid metabolism. Glycosphingolipids are normal constituents of the plasma membrane as well as the membranes of intracellular organelles. In Fabry disease, the α-Gal A deficiency results in a tissue accumulation of trihexosylceramide causing the disease's systemic manifestations [1]. Early and often asymptomatic cellular damage typically precedes various degrees of organ affection that can lead to progressive organ failure [2]. Males with less than 1% α-Gal A enzyme activity usually present with classic Fabry disease characterized by onset in childhood or adolescence. Symptoms include acroparesthesia, angiokeratomas, hypohidrosis or anhidrosis, characteristic corneal and lenticular opacities, cardiac disease, cerebrovascular manifestations, proteinuria, and gradual deterioration of renal function, as well as gastrointestinal, auditory, pulmonary, vascular, and psychological manifestations [4–12]. Males with greater than 1% α-Gal A activity may have later-onset phenotypes and typically develop renal and/or cardiac disease in their fourth to seventh decades of life [13, 14]. Heterozygous females usually have milder symptoms and a later age of onset than males. However, there is broad phenotypic variability and they may have symptoms as severe as those observed in males with the classic form [15, 16], possibly due to skewed X-chromosome inactivation [1, 17].

To date, more than 1000 mutations in the *GLA* gene have been identified [18], and research on clinically relevant genotype-phenotype relationships is increasingly prioritized [2]. Most of the pathogenic *GLA* mutations are private, occurring in a single or few families; intra-familial phenotypic variability has been observed, complicating the study of genotype-phenotype correlations [19]. Some mutations can be associated with the classic phenotype that includes nonsense, most of the splicing and frameshift mutations resulting in little or no α-Gal A enzyme activity [19]. In contrast, some missense mutations can encode enzymes with residual α-Gal A activity presenting with the later-onset phenotypes [19–21].

Current therapeutic approaches for Fabry disease include the reduction of accumulated glycosphingolipids through enzyme-replacement therapy (ERT) and a pharmacological chaperone for a subset of Fabry patients with amenable mutations, along with symptomatic and palliative treatments when needed [22]. In this chapter, we will focus on ERT in Fabry disease, which has clearly demonstrated a modifying effect on serious organ complications and mortality. Kidney manifestations in Fabry disease and the effect of ERT on clinical nephrological outcomes will be highlighted.

2. Kidney manifestations in Fabry disease

Nephropathy caused by intracellular accumulation of globotriaosylceramide (Gb3) in the kidney, is one of the main features of Fabry disease. Kidney manifestations occur in at least 50% of male patients and approximately 20% of female patients [16]. A urinary concentration defect, microalbuminuria, and later overt proteinuria and progressive decline of kidney function are important signs of Fabry nephropathy [23].

2.1 Proteinuria

Proteinuria is the most important biomarker in Fabry nephropathy. Studies showed urinary protein excretion is strongly associated with renal disease progression in men and women with Fabry disease [24]. Proteinuria may be glomerular or tubular in origin and usually appears during the second to third decades of life in affected individuals [23, 25, 26]. Early-onset of proteinuria is not rare and it has been reported in male and female adolescents and in boys as young as 6 years [23]. Approximately 90% of males with Fabry disease developed proteinuria by the age of 50 years [27]. Approximately 30–35% of females with Fabry disease have overt proteinuria with an age of onset that is usually later than in males [27–29]. Though proteinuria is an early complication of renal injury, it may not be overt in some patients even with advanced kidney disease [28].

The mechanism of proteinuria has not been entirely clear. Gb3 deposits in podocytes have not been directly related to the magnitude of proteinuria [23]. The degree of proteinuria is a major prognostic determinant for more rapidly progressive Fabry nephropathy, particularly in adult male patients, and may also directly contribute to the progression of renal disease [23].

Nephrotic-range proteinuria is uncommon. In a long-term natural history study from the National Institutes of Health (NIH), nephrotic proteinuria was found in 18% of patients with renal disease. The age at onset of nephrotic proteinuria was 40 ± 7 years (range 26–55 yr). The full presentation of nephrotic syndrome was uncommon even in patients who had heavy proteinuria [27].

2.2 Renal tubular dysfunction

Gb3 accumulation in the kidney occurs in all renal cells but preferentially in the glomeruli, distal tubular cells, and vascular smooth muscle cells. Injury of distal tubular cells leads to urinary concentration defects presenting with polyuria, nocturia, and polydipsia, which may be the early signs of Fabry kidney disease [27, 30]. Interestingly, one case report has suggested that screening for mulberry cells (regarded as distal tubular epithelial cells in which Gb3 has accumulated) during urinalysis could be a simple, inexpensive, and noninvasive method for diagnosing Fabry nephropathy in the absence of proteinuria [31, 32]. Gb3 deposition in proximal tubules may rarely lead to proximal renal tubular acidosis or even Fanconi syndrome. The urine sediment in Fabry disease may contain oval fat bodies, which are renal tubular epithelial cells or cell fragments with lipid inclusions. Under microscopy using crossed polarization filters, these oval fat bodies demonstrate a typical Maltese cross configuration with a lamellar appearance [27].

2.3 Chronic kidney disease

Initially, patients with Fabry disease may have glomerular hyperfiltration at a rate similar to diabetic nephropathy [23, 33]. However, when the number of damaged nephrons reaches a critical level that cannot maintain adequate glomerular filtration, there will be a rapid decline in GFR [23]. CKD is prevalent in untreated patients with Fabry disease and typically progresses to end-stage renal disease (ESRD). In a cross-sectional retrospective analysis of the natural history of glomerular filtration rate (estimated-eGFR), albuminuria, and proteinuria in 1262 adult patients (585 males, 677 females) using data from the Fabry Registry before treatment with ERT, chronic kidney disease (CKD) stages 1 or 2 were found in 72% of males and 87% of females. CKD with eGFR <60 ml/min/1.73 m [2] was found in 28% of males and 13% of females, while in patients aged >40 years, the percentage increased to 45 and 20% [28]. Without ERT, progression rates of renal insufficiency can be as high as seen in diabetic nephropathy [23]. In the NIH series described above, 39 of 105 patients developed CKD defined as a serum creatinine concentration ≥ 1.5 mg/dL, and the median age of CKD onset and ESRD was 42 years and 47 years, respectively, with a time of progression from onset of CKD to ESRD 4 ± 3 years (range 1–13 yr) [27].

2.4 Hypertension

Hypertension is not a common early finding in patients with Fabry disease but becomes more prevalent with disease progression [23]. In the NIH series, hypertension was present in 31 patients (30%) with onset at age 38 ± 11 years (range 14–54 yr). Thirty-five percent of patients developed hypertension before the onset of CKD, 12% of patients had a simultaneous diagnosis of hypertension and CKD, and 53% of patients developed hypertension 5 ± 5 years after the onset of CKD [27], suggesting that the onset of CKD was followed by the development of hypertension in most patients.

2.5 Renal sinus and parapelvic cysts

Renal cysts are common, particularly in older men. Studies from potential living kidney donors showed that a cortical, medullary, or parapelvic cyst ≥5 mm was present in 12%, 14%, and 2.8%, respectively [34]. Renal sinus and parapelvic cysts are more prevalent in patients with Fabry disease compared to the general population and are considered as a distinguishing feature in Fabry disease [35]. In a cross-sectional case-control study with 24 patients affected with classic Fabry disease (mean age 36.1 ± 8.1 years, median 37 years, range 20–48 years), prospective renal imaging evaluation with magnetic resonance imaging (MRI) and computed tomography (CT) showed 50% of Fabry disease patients had renal sinus cysts, compared to one individual (7%) in the control group [35]. The etiology and mechanism of sinus cyst formation in Fabry disease remain unclear.

2.6 Renal pathology

Renal biopsy is important not only for confirming the diagnosis, but also to show renal damage that can occur in some patients with minimal or no evidence of renal disease on standard tests [23]. By light microscopy, the cells, especially podocytes, parietal epithelial cells, and distal tubular epithelial cells, appear vacuolated because the accumulated glycosphingolipid inclusions are removed during tissue processing for paraffin embedding. Hyaline-like material accumulates in the media of arteries and arterioles and sometimes in the mesangial regions [36]. Immunofluorescence is typically negative. By electron microscopy, podocytes are filled with osmiophilic, granular-to-lamellated membrane structures (zebra bodies) [23, 27, 36].

3. Enzyme-replacement therapy (ERT)

Before ERT was available, a reduced life span of about 25 years in males and 10 years in females was expected compared with the general population [2, 37]. Clinical research with follow-up data clearly demonstrates a modifying effect of ERT on serious organ complications and mortality. ERT has been available for the treatment of Fabry disease since 2001 in Europe and since 2003 in the USA. Licensed ERT treatments include agalsidase alfa (Replagal™, Shire Human Genetic Therapies/Takeda Pharmaceuticals Europe Ltd., London, UK), agalsidase beta (Fabrazyme™, Sanofi Genzyme, Cambridge, MA), and agalsidase beta biosimilar (Fabagal™, Isu-Abxis, South Korea). Agalsidase beta is licensed in both the USA and Europe, while agalsidase alfa is not licensed in the USA. Fabagal is approved in South Korea [22]. Agalsidase alfa is produced in a genetically engineered human cell line and agalsidase beta is produced in a Chinese hamster ovary cell line [38].

4. Efficacy of ERT

In a 20-week multicenter, randomized, placebo-controlled, double-blind phase 3 clinical trial of 58 patients who were at least 16 years old and had enzymatically confirmed classic Fabry disease, agalsidase beta at 1 mg/kg/2 weeks cleared microvascular endothelial deposits of Gb3 from the kidneys, heart, and skin, reversing the chief clinical manifestation of this disease [39].

Further investigation was performed to analyze the pre- and post-treatment renal biopsies from these Fabry disease patients and the authors found that after 11 months of ERT, complete clearance of glycolipid storage was noted from the endothelium of all vasculature, the mesangial cells of the glomerulus, and interstitial cells of the cortex, while moderate clearance was noted from the smooth muscle cells of arterioles and small arteries [40]. Limited clearance of glycolipid storage was also observed from podocytes and distal tubular epithelium [40].

An open-label, phase 3 extension study was conducted involving these 58 patients who completed the 20-week study and were transitioned to an extension trial to receive agalsidase beta biweekly at 1 mg/kg for up to an additional 54 months [41]. Authors reported by month 54 all assessable patients maintained clearance of glycolipid storage clearance from multiple renal cell types, including renal capillary endothelial cells, mesangial cells, and noncapillary endothelial cells. Sustained clearance of skin and heart capillary endothelium was also demonstrated by month 54. Mean plasma Gb3 levels remained controlled in the normal range and kidney function remained stable in patients with data available. This study suggested baseline proteinuria (>1 g/24 h), >50% glomerulosclerosis, and age > 40 years at treatment baseline as important factors that limited renal response to therapy [41].

Furthermore, a study was conducted to investigate the long-term outcomes in 52 of these 58 patients including severe clinical events, renal function, and cardiac structure following treatment with agalsidase beta (1 mg/kg/2 weeks) over a 10-year median follow-up period. Authors reported that 81% of patients (42/52) did not experience any severe clinical event during the treatment interval and 94% (49/52) were alive at the end of the study period [17]. Mean slopes for eGFR for low renal involvement and high renal involvement were −1.89 mL/min/1.73 m^2/year and −6.82 mL/min/1.73 m^2/year, respectively [17]. Patients with low renal involvement started therapy 13 years younger than those with high renal involvement. This 10-year study documented the effectiveness of agalsidase beta (1 mg/kg/2 weeks) in patients with Fabry disease and suggested patients who initiated treatment at a younger age and with less kidney involvement benefited the most from therapy [17].

In addition, a recent meta-analysis with the evidence base including four Sanofi Genzyme studies and six studies from a systematic literature review suggested that treated (agalsidase beta) patients experienced a slower median eGFR decrease [2.46 mL/min/1.73 m^2/year slower; 95% confidence interval (CI) 0.63–4.29; P ¼ 0.0087] than comparable untreated patients [22].

5. Initiation of ERT

Initiation of ERT requires a fully confirmed diagnosis of Fabry disease [19]. The patient/patient's family should be included in the decision-making process and should have a good understanding of the impact of the treatment as well as potential adverse reactions. The initiation of lifelong ERT infusion therapy is a major decision with important implications for both the patient, particularly the pediatric patient, and the family [42]. Treatment and follow-up assessments should ideally be led by a physician who is experienced in the management of patients with Fabry disease, with support from a multidisciplinary clinical team including nephrology, cardiology, medical genetics, neurology, psychology, and nursing [19].

5.1 Adult Fabry patients

As indicated in the clinical studies above, early initiation of ERT seemed associated with more clinical benefits. For adult patients, in our practice, we follow the expert guideline from an international panel of Fabry disease experts from multiple subspecialties published in 2018 [19] and outlined below:

- For all adult male patients with *GLA* variants consistent with classic Fabry disease, ERT should be initiated regardless of Fabry symptoms [19].

- For adult symptomatic female patients with *GLA* variants consistent with classic Fabry disease and clinical signs/symptoms suggesting major organ involvement, initiation of ERT should be considered. The signs/symptoms include proteinuria/albuminuria not attributable to other causes, evidence of renal impairment (may require renal biopsy if isolated); stroke or TIA; neuropathic pain, pain crises, Fabry disease neuropathy; symptomatic cardiac disease not due to other causes (dyspnea, palpitations, syncope, chest pain); exercise intolerance and impaired sweating; recurrent diarrhea, chronic, disabling GI dysfunction (excluding alternative causes) [19].

- For adult, asymptomatic female patients with *GLA* variants consistent with classic Fabry disease with laboratory, histological, or imaging evidence of injury to the kidney, heart, or the CNS, ERT should be also considered. The evidence includes decreased GFR (< 90 mL/min/1.73 m [2] adjusted for age > 40 years), persistent albuminuria >30 mg/g, renal biopsy proved podocyte foot process effacement or glomerulosclerosis, moderate or severe Gb3 inclusions in a range of renal cell types; silent strokes, cerebral white matter lesions on brain MRI; asymptomatic cardiac disease including cardiomyopathy, arrhythmia, or cardiac fibrosis on contrast cardiac MRI. Predominant expression of the mutant *GLA* allele is generally associated with rapid disease progression, requiring closer monitoring and early therapeutic intervention. If a skewed X-chromosome inactivation pattern with predominant expression of the mutant *GLA* allele has been demonstrated in the presence of signs and symptoms of disease, experts suggested ERT should also be considered [19].

- For adult male and female patients with *GLA* variants consistent with later-onset Fabry disease or missense *GLA* variants of unknown significance (VUS), experts suggest ERT should be considered and is appropriate if there is a laboratory, histological, or imaging evidence of injury to the kidney, heart, or the CNS attributable to Fabry disease, even in the absence of typical Fabry symptoms. The interpretation of the pathogenicity of any VUS should involve an expert in genetics and management of Fabry disease. Individuals with well-characterized benign *GLA* polymorphisms should not be treated with ERT [19]. For patients without Fabry disease-related tissue pathology or clinical symptoms, particularly heterozygous female patients, some experts suggested a "wait and watch" approach to monitor patients regularly by a multidisciplinary care team [19].

5.2 Pediatric Fabry patients

In the pediatric population, renal damage is typically subclinical and identifiable only through biopsy. In young patients with Fabry disease, timely initiation of ERT is important because some early pathological changes are potentially reversible by ERT [42, 43]. As discussed above, the 10-year study of the effectiveness of agalsidase beta in patients with classic Fabry disease has demonstrated that adults who initiated treatment at a younger age and with less renal involvement benefited more from therapy [17, 42]. Therefore, early diagnosis of patients with Fabry disease is vital for appropriate management and monitoring. In our practice, we follow the consensus guideline developed by specialists from the United States with expertise in Fabry disease about the management and treatment of children with Fabry disease [42], which has considerable overlap but also some differences compared to the recommendations by the European Fabry Working Group [44].

- For symptomatic boys and girls, the experts in the United States recommended treatment with ERT should be considered and is appropriate if Fabry symptoms are present at any age [42]. Symptomatic girls and boys should be treated and managed in the same way, with the goal of decreasing symptomatology and reducing the risk of disease progression [42]. These recommendations are similar to those by the European Fabry Working Group [44]. Girls with Fabry disease commonly develop nonspecific early symptoms, such as abdominal pain, diarrhea, and neuropathic pain, around the age of 9–10 years [42, 45]. These symptoms should be considered adequate evidence of progressive disease to recommend the initiation of ERT [42].

- For asymptomatic boys with *GLA* variants consistent with classic Fabry disease, experts in the United States recommend the timing of ERT depending on the individual case, carefully balancing the risks and benefits of therapy. Clinicians should have a serious discussion with the family to consider initiation of ERT by age 8–10 years [42]. This consensus recommendation was reached based on data from renal biopsy studies and responses to ERT that noted the greater difficulty in initiating infusions in children younger than this age [42]. These United States consensus recommendations do not concur with the European Fabry Working Group recommendations for treatment initiation at 16 years [42, 44].

- For asymptomatic girls and asymptomatic boys with late-onset variants or VUS, the decision to defer ERT should be based on comprehensive longitudinal monitoring for the development of clinical symptoms and signs of disease. The family history of the female patients should also be considered [42].

5.3 Dosing and duration of therapy

As mentioned above, the two widely used forms of ERT for Fabry disease are agalsidase alfa and agalsidase beta and there have not been any trials comparing these formulations to one another [46].

The formulations of agalsidase alfa and agalsidase beta are structurally very similar to one another [47–49], however, they are not dosed the same. Agalsidase alfa is dosed at 0.2 mg/kg every other week [50],while agalsidase beta is dosed at 1.0 mg/kg every other week [51]. For patients who weigh less than 30 kg, the infusion rate of agalsidase beta should not exceed 15 mg/hr.

There are no clinical trials to determine the duration of ERT [52] in patients that meet the criteria to be treated, however, treatment is generally continued until a reason for stopping therapy arises. The most agreed-upon reasons for stopping therapy are noncompliance with infusions, failure to attend regular follow up visits, end-stage Fabry disease or other co-morbidities leading to a life expectancy of

<1 year, lack of response for 1 year when the sole indication for ERT is neuropathic pain while receiving maximum supportive care, or persistent life-threatening or severe reactions that do not respond to prophylaxis and patient request [44].

The Fabry registry website includes a detailed table resource that can be used as a visual to guide a prescriber on what lab values, imaging, and other studies should be monitored, specifically in the pediatric population. This can be found in the Fabry Registry section entitled "Fabry Registry Recommended Schedule of Assessments." The page can be found using the following web address:

https://www.fabrydisease.org/images/ReferencePDFs/fabry-registry-schedule-of-assessments.pdf

5.4 Side effects and what to monitor in patients receiving ERT

The side effects of ERT that were mentioned in the early trials included side effects that are common with infusions including fevers and rigors. These infusion-associated reactions are often treated prophylactically with antihistamines, acetaminophen, and pre-infusion steroids sometimes becoming necessary. It is not uncommon that lengthening of infusion times becomes necessary because of these reactions [39, 50]. There have been reported life-threatening infusion-associated reactions, although those are rare [53].

Expert recommendations have been used to determine potential scheduled assessment and monitoring. The patient will undergo the most amount of testing upon initial evaluation including a full medical history (including family history, physical examination, vital signs, and quality of life), basic metabolic panel, urine protein excretion, lipid panels, and other measures for cardiac, cerebrovascular, neurological, ENT, pulmonary, and ophthalmological assessments. Plasma samples for Gb3 testing should be drawn prior to the first infusion, then every 3 months for the first 18 months of treatment, then every 6 months thereafter. It is reasonable to do a monitoring of serum chemistries and a complete blood count every 6–12 months in all patients. In patients with kidney disease, consider monitoring urinary protein excretion every 3 months. All patients regardless of renal involvement should have annual urinary protein measurement. A baseline kidney biopsy can serve as a potential marker to assess disease progression if the patient experiences deterioration of his/her condition and a repeat biopsy is warranted [19].

The formation of neutralizing antidrug antibodies (ADAs) is not uncommon in patients with Fabry disease receiving ERT [50, 54, 55]. These antibodies are associated with increased accumulation of plasma globotriaosylceramide and disease progression [56]. An open cohort study showed ADA titers decreased significantly in all patients with Fabry disease during ERT infusion and that a not saturated ADA status during infusion is associated with progressive loss of eGFR and ongoing cardiac hypertrophy. Dose escalation can result in saturation of ADAs and decreasing Gb3 levels but may lead to increased ADA titers [56]. Immunosuppression may be considered should ADAs develop but it is not clear how much long-term protection it can offer. Serum samples for IgG antibody testing should be drawn prior to the first infusion, then every 3 months for the first 18 months of treatment, then every 6 months until two consecutive negative results are confirmed.

5.5 Creating a protocol in the infusion center

Patients with Fabry disease need ERT infusions every other week. The information needed for drug administration often comes from the manufacturer. The information we supply here is for agalsidase beta and serves as an example of what kind of resources would be needed to create a protocol and provide this medication at an infusion center.

Agalsidase beta comes in 5 mg and 35 mg vials that are initially injected with sterile water to create a colorless solution. This solution is then further diluted with 0.9% sodium chloride that is diluted to a higher volume, which is supplied by the manufacturer. Once the diluted solution is created, it is recommended that it be used immediately. If that is not possible, the solution can be stored for 24 h at a temperature of 2–8°C. The initial infusion rate of the solution should be no more than 15 mg/h and this can be slowed down further for infusion-associated reactions. For patients that weigh >30 kg and after the infusion is well-tolerated, the infusion rate can be increased by 3–5 mg/h with each infusion. The minimal infusion time for patients >30 kg should be 1.5 h.

Antipyretics are recommended to be administered prior to the enzymatic infusion. If a patient experiences an infusion-associated reaction, options include decreasing the infusion rate, temporarily stopping the infusion, and/or administering additional antipyretics, antihistamines, and/or steroids if needed. Prophylactic antihistamines and/or steroids can be considered in patients who experience infusion-related reactions. Life-threatening anaphylactic reactions can occur and require immediate discontinuation of the infusion as well as a center that is equipped with appropriate medical support measures and the capability to handle such scenarios.

5.6 Cost

ERT is expensive. The estimated retail cost of therapy with Fabrazyme for 1 year is approximately USD 300,000 in the United States and Europe.

6. Summary

In short, Fabry disease is a multi-systemic disease associated with a high burden of morbidity and mortality.

The clinical outcome of patients with Fabry disease has drastically changed with the introduction of ERT. Timely initiation of ERT and regular assessments of disease progression by a multidisciplinary care team are critical for the long-term management of patients with Fabry disease.

Author details

Hanny Sawaf[1], Angelika L. Erwin[2], Fang Zhao[3], Tushar J. Vachharajani[1] and Xiangling Wang[1,2,4]*

1 Department of Kidney Medicine, Glickman Urology and Kidney Institute, Cleveland, Ohio, USA

2 Center for Personalized Genetic Healthcare, Cleveland Clinic Community Care and Population Health, Cleveland, Ohio, USA

3 Department of Pathology, The Center of Clinical Informatics Research and Education, Metrohealth System/Case Western Reserve University, Cleveland, Ohio, USA

4 Molecular Medicine, Cleveland Clinic Lerner College of Medicine of Case Western Reserve University, Cleveland, Ohio, USA

*Address all correspondence to: wangx8@ccf.org

References

[1] Germain DP. Fabry disease. Orphanet Journal of Rare Diseases. 2010;**5**:30

[2] Svarstad E, Marti HP. The changing landscape of Fabry disease. Clinical Journal of the American Society of Nephrology. 2020;**15**:569-576

[3] Meikle PJ, Hopwood JJ, Clague AE, Carey WF. Prevalence of lysosomal storage disorders. Journal of the American Medical Association. 1999;**281**:249-254

[4] Hegemann S, Hajioff D, Conti G, Beck M, Sunder-Plassmann G, Widmer U, et al. Hearing loss in Fabry disease: Data from the Fabry Outcome Survey. European Journal of Clinical Investigation. 2006;**36**:654-662

[5] Orteu CH, Jansen T, Lidove O, Jaussaud R, Hughes DA, Pintos-Morell G, et al. Fabry disease and the skin: Data from FOS, the Fabry outcome survey. The British Journal of Dermatology. 2007;**157**:331-337

[6] Lidove O, Ramaswami U, Jaussaud R, Barbey F, Maisonobe T, Caillaud C, et al. Hyperhidrosis: A new and often early symptom in Fabry disease. International experience and data from the Fabry Outcome Survey. International Journal of Clinical Practise. 2006;**60**:1053-1059

[7] Sodi A, Ioannidis AS, Mehta A, Davey C, Beck M, Pitz S. Ocular manifestations of Fabry's disease: Data from the Fabry Outcome Survey. The British Journal of Ophthalmology. 2007;**91**:210-214

[8] Linhart A, Kampmann C, Zamorano JL, Sunder-Plassmann G, Beck M, Mehta A, et al. Cardiac manifestations of Anderson-Fabry disease: Results from the international Fabry outcome survey. European Heart Journal. 2007;**28**:1228-1235

[9] Politei JM, Capizzano AA. Magnetic resonance image findings in 5 young patients with Fabry disease. The Neurologist. 2006;**12**:103-105

[10] Hoffmann B, Schwarz M, Mehta A, Keshav S, Fabry Outcome Survey European I. Gastrointestinal symptoms in 342 patients with Fabry disease: Prevalence and response to enzyme replacement therapy. Clinical Gastroenterology and Hepatology. 2007;**5**:1447-1453

[11] Magage S, Lubanda JC, Susa Z, Bultas J, Karetova D, Dobrovolny R, et al. Natural history of the respiratory involvement in Anderson-Fabry disease. Journal of Inherited Metabolic Disease. 2007;**30**:790-799

[12] Cole AL, Lee PJ, Hughes DA, Deegan PB, Waldek S, Lachmann RH. Depression in adults with Fabry disease: A common and under-diagnosed problem. Journal of Inherited Metabolic Disease. 2007;**30**:943-951

[13] Patel V, O'Mahony C, Hughes D, Rahman MS, Coats C, Murphy E, et al. Clinical and genetic predictors of major cardiac events in patients with Anderson-Fabry Disease. Heart. 2015;**101**:961-966

[14] Nakao S, Kodama C, Takenaka T, Tanaka A, Yasumoto Y, Yoshida A, et al. Fabry disease: Detection of undiagnosed hemodialysis patients and identification of a "renal variant" phenotype. Kidney International. 2003;**64**:801-807

[15] Gupta S, Ries M, Kotsopoulos S, Schiffmann R. The relationship of vascular glycolipid storage to clinical manifestations of Fabry disease: A cross-sectional study of a large cohort of clinically affected heterozygous women. Medicine (Baltimore). 2005;**84**:261-268

[16] Wilcox WR, Oliveira JP, Hopkin RJ, Ortiz A, Banikazemi M,

Feldt-Rasmussen U, et al. Females with Fabry disease frequently have major organ involvement: Lessons from the Fabry Registry. Molecular Genetics and Metabolism. 2008;**93**:112-128

[17] Germain DP, Charrow J, Desnick RJ, Guffon N, Kempf J, Lachmann RH, et al. Ten-year outcome of enzyme replacement therapy with agalsidase beta in patients with Fabry disease. Journal of Medical Genetics. 2015;**52**:353-358

[18] Kurschat CE. Fabry disease-what cardiologists can learn from the nephrologist: A narrative review. Cardiovascular Diagnosos and Therapy. 2021;**11**:672-682

[19] Ortiz A, Germain DP, Desnick RJ, Politei J, Mauer M, Burlina A, et al. Fabry disease revisited: Management and treatment recommendations for adult patients. Molecular Genetics and Metabolism. 2018;**123**:416-427

[20] Schaefer E, Mehta A, Gal A. Genotype and phenotype in Fabry disease: Analysis of the Fabry Outcome Survey. Acta Paediatrica. 2005;**94**:87-92

[21] Schafer E, Baron K, Widmer U, Deegan P, Neumann HP, Sunder-Plassmann G, et al. Thirty-four novel mutations of the GLA gene in 121 patients with Fabry disease. Human Mutation. 2005;**25**:412

[22] Ortiz A, Kanters S, Hamed A, DasMahapatra P, Poggio E, Maski M, et al. Agalsidase beta treatment slows estimated glomerular filtration rate loss in classic Fabry disease patients: Results from an individual patient data meta-analysis. Clinical Kidney Journal. 2021;**14**:1136-1146

[23] Torra R. Renal manifestations in Fabry disease and therapeutic options. Kidney International. 2008;**Suppl 111**: S29-S32

[24] Wanner C, Oliveira JP, Ortiz A, Mauer M, Germain DP, Linthorst GE, et al. Prognostic indicators of renal disease progression in adults with Fabry disease: Natural history data from the Fabry Registry. Clinical Journal of the American Society of Nephrology. 2010;**5**:2220-2228

[25] Eng CM, Fletcher J, Wilcox WR, Waldek S, Scott CR, Sillence DO, et al. Fabry disease: Baseline medical characteristics of a cohort of 1765 males and females in the Fabry Registry. Journal of Inherited Metabolic Disease. 2007;**30**:184-192

[26] Mehta A, Ricci R, Widmer U, Dehout F, Garcia de Lorenzo A, Kampmann C, et al. Fabry disease defined: Baseline clinical manifestations of 366 patients in the Fabry Outcome Survey. European Journal of Clinical Investigation. 2004;**34**:236-242

[27] Branton MH, Schiffmann R, Sabnis SG, Murray GJ, Quirk JM, Altarescu G, et al. Natural history of Fabry renal disease: Influence of alpha-galactosidase A activity and genetic mutations on clinical course. Medicine (Baltimore). 2002; **81**:122-138

[28] Ortiz A, Oliveira JP, Waldek S, Warnock DG, Cianciaruso B, Wanner C, et al. Nephropathy in males and females with Fabry disease: Cross-sectional description of patients before treatment with enzyme replacement therapy. Nephrology, Dialysis, Transplantation. 2008;**23**:1600-1607

[29] Deegan PB, Baehner AF, Barba Romero MA, Hughes DA, Kampmann C, Beck M, et al. Natural history of Fabry disease in females in the Fabry Outcome Survey. Journal of Medical Genetics. 2006;**43**:347-352

[30] Branton M, Schiffmann R, Kopp JB. Natural history and treatment of renal involvement in Fabry disease. Journal of

American Social Nephrology. 2002;**13**(Suppl 2):S139-S143

[31] Del Pino M, Andres A, Bernabeu AA, de Juan-Rivera J, Fernandez E, de Dios Garcia Diaz J, et al. Fabry nephropathy: An evidence-based narrative review. Kidney & Blood Pressure Research. 2018;**43**:406-421

[32] Nakamichi T, Miyazaki M, Nakayama K, Sato M, Akiu N, Sato T, et al. Fabry's disease discovered with chance urinary mulberry cells: A case report. CEN Case Reports. 2013;**2**:49-52

[33] Sessa A, Meroni M, Battini G, Righetti M, Maglio A, Tosoni A, et al. Renal involvement in Anderson-Fabry disease. Journal of Nephrology. 2003;**16**:310-313

[34] Rule AD, Sasiwimonphan K, Lieske JC, Keddis MT, Torres VE, Vrtiska TJ. Characteristics of renal cystic and solid lesions based on contrast-enhanced computed tomography of potential kidney donors. American Journal of Kidney Diseases. 2012;**59**:611-618

[35] Ries M, Bettis KE, Choyke P, Kopp JB, Austin HA 3rd, Brady RO, et al. Parapelvic kidney cysts: A distinguishing feature with high prevalence in Fabry disease. Kidney International. 2004;**66**:978-982

[36] Najafian B, Fogo AB, Lusco MA, Alpers CE. AJKD atlas of renal pathology: Fabry nephropathy. American Journal of Kidney Diseases. 2015;**66**:e35-e36

[37] Schiffmann R, Warnock DG, Banikazemi M, Bultas J, Linthorst GE, Packman S, et al. Fabry disease: Progression of nephropathy, and prevalence of cardiac and cerebrovascular events before enzyme replacement therapy. Nephrology, Dialysis, Transplantation. 2009;**24**:2102-2111

[38] Lubanda JC, Anijalg E, Bzduch V, Thurberg BL, Benichou B, Tylki-Szymanska A. Evaluation of a low dose, after a standard therapeutic dose, of agalsidase beta during enzyme replacement therapy in patients with Fabry disease. Genetics in Medicine. 2009;**11**:256-264

[39] Eng CM, Guffon N, Wilcox WR, Germain DP, Lee P, Waldek S, et al. Safety and efficacy of recombinant human alpha-galactosidase A replacement therapy in Fabry's disease. The New England Journal of Medicine. 2001;**345**:9-16

[40] Thurberg BL, Rennke H, Colvin RB, Dikman S, Gordon RE, Collins AB, et al. Globotriaosylceramide accumulation in the Fabry kidney is cleared from multiple cell types after enzyme replacement therapy. Kidney International. 2002;**62**:1933-1946

[41] Germain DP, Waldek S, Banikazemi M, Bushinsky DA, Charrow J, Desnick RJ, et al. Sustained, long-term renal stabilization after 54 months of agalsidase beta therapy in patients with Fabry disease. Journal of American Social Nephrology. 2007;**18**:1547-1557

[42] Hopkin RJ, Jefferies JL, Laney DA, Lawson VH, Mauer M, Taylor MR, et al. The management and treatment of children with Fabry disease: A United States-based perspective. Molecular Genetics Metabolism. 2016; **117**:104-113

[43] Tondel C, Bostad L, Larsen KK, Hirth A, Vikse BE, Houge G, et al. Agalsidase benefits renal histology in young patients with Fabry disease. Journal of American Social Nephrology. 2013;**24**:137-148

[44] Biegstraaten M, Arngrimsson R, Barbey F, Boks L, Cecchi F, Deegan PB, et al. Recommendations for initiation and cessation of enzyme replacement

therapy in patients with Fabry disease: The European Fabry Working Group consensus document. Orphanet Journal of Rare Diseases. 2015;**10**:36

[45] Hopkin RJ, Bissler J, Banikazemi M, Clarke L, Eng CM, Germain DP, et al. Characterization of Fabry disease in 352 pediatric patients in the Fabry Registry. Pediatric Research. 2008;**64**:550-555

[46] El Dib R, Gomaa H, Carvalho RP, Camargo SE, Bazan R, Barretti P, et al. Enzyme replacement therapy for Anderson-Fabry disease. Cochrane Database of Systematic Reviews. 2016;**7**:CD006663

[47] Lee K, Jin X, Zhang K, Copertino L, Andrews L, Baker-Malcolm J, et al. A biochemical and pharmacological comparison of enzyme replacement therapies for the glycolipid storage disorder Fabry disease. Glycobiology. 2003;**13**:305-313

[48] Blom D, Speijer D, Linthorst GE, Donker-Koopman WG, Strijland A, Aerts JM. Recombinant enzyme therapy for Fabry disease: Absence of editing of human alpha-galactosidase A mRNA. American Journal of Human Genetics. 2003;**72**:23-31

[49] Sakuraba H, Murata-Ohsawa M, Kawashima I, Tajima Y, Kotani M, Ohshima T, et al. Comparison of the effects of agalsidase alfa and agalsidase beta on cultured human Fabry fibroblasts and Fabry mice. Journal of Human Genetics. 2006;**51**:180-188

[50] Schiffmann R, Kopp JB, Austin HA 3rd, Sabnis S, Moore DF, Weibel T, et al. Enzyme replacement therapy in Fabry disease: A randomized controlled trial. Journal of the American Medical Association. 2001;**285**:2743-2749

[51] Lenders M, Stypmann J, Duning T, Schmitz B, Brand SM, Brand E. Serum-mediated inhibition of enzyme replacement therapy in Fabry disease. Journal of American Society of Nephrology. 2016;**27**:256-264

[52] Germain DP, Elliott PM, Falissard B, Fomin VV, Hilz MJ, Jovanovic A, et al. The effect of enzyme replacement therapy on clinical outcomes in male patients with Fabry disease: A systematic literature review by a European panel of experts. Molecular Genetetics of Metabolic Reports. 2019;**19**:100454

[53] Nicholls K, Bleasel K, Becker G. Severe infusion reactions to fabry enzyme replacement therapy: Rechallenge after tracheostomy. JIMD Reports. 2012;**5**:109-112

[54] Lidove O, West ML, Pintos-Morell G, Reisin R, Nicholls K, Figuera LE, et al. Effects of enzyme replacement therapy in Fabry disease: A comprehensive review of the medical literature. Genetics in Medicine. 2010;**12**:668-679

[55] Banikazemi M, Bultas J, Waldek S, Wilcox WR, Whitley CB, McDonald M, et al. Agalsidase-beta therapy for advanced Fabry disease: A randomized trial. Annals of Internal Medicine. 2007;**146**:77-86

[56] Lenders M, Neusser LP, Rudnicki M, Nordbeck P, Canaan-Kuhl S, Nowak A, et al. Dose-dependent effect of enzyme replacement therapy on neutralizing antidrug antibody titers and clinical outcome in patients with Fabry disease. Journal of American Society of Nephrology. 2018;**29**:2879-2889

Chapter 8

Prognostic Value of Serum Parathyroid Hormone in Patients with End-Stage Renal Disease

Raid D. Hashim

Abstract

End-stage renal disease (ESRD) is a clinical condition related to prolonged and irreversible loss of renal function. In addition to many others, it is associated with various disorders of calcium, magnesium and phosphorus metabolism which usually appears early in the course of the condition. Secondary hyperparathyroidism is a characteristic finding in patients with ESRD secondary to the previously mentioned metabolic abnormalities. The associated increase in plasma level of parathyroid hormone (PTH) has been correlated to many complications that accompany ESRD. These conditions might represent the major cause of mortality in certain circumstances. In light of this suggested impact of plasma level of PTH on many complications that are usually present in patients with ESRD, it might be of great benefit to regularly test this hormone in such patients.

Keywords: parathyroid hormone, end-stage-renal- disease, hypocalcemia, hyperphosphatemia, hemodialysis

1. Introduction

Calcium is one of the essential minerals in the human body being enrolled in various metabolic functions. About 99% of the total body's calcium is present in bone, but the remaining fraction that is present in plasma or the intracellular compartment has a vital role in muscular contraction, normal blood coagulation system, cardiac muscle contractility and rhythm in addition to many other vital functions. Calcium homeostasis requires integration among various organs within the human body such as parathyroid glands, intestine and kidneys. In other words, normal concentration of plasma parathyroid hormone, intact absorptive function of the intestine, proper activation of vitamin D and normal renal re-absorptive and excretory function are all essential to maintain plasma calcium level within the reference range. In patients with chronic kidney disease (CKD), specifically those with advanced stage, there will be an associated progressive impairment of vitamin D activation due to progressive loss of nephrons. This will lead to significant malabsorption of calcium by the intestine with consequent hypocalcemia. This hypocalcemia, in addition to other factors, represents a major stimulus on parathyroid hormone (PTH) secretion by one of two mechanisms that are dependent on the duration of hypocalcemia. In the short term, hypocalcemia will stimulate PTH secretion via G-protein while prolonged hypocalcemia is associated with altered stability of m-RNA-encoding PTH. The pathophysiology of hypocalcemia in patients with chronic kidney disease is related to two main factors. First, the precipitation of calcium on various body tissues after being complexed with plasma phosphorus that is present in higher concentrations. Second, impaired absorption of calcium at the intestine secondary to the deficient active form of the vitamin (1,25 (OH)2 vitamin D) due to improper activation of vitamin D by the renal cortex. Because of the prolonged stimulation of parathyroid glands by the persistent hypocalcemia in patients with chronic kidney disease, secondary hyperparathyroidism will be an expected associated finding in such patients. So, secondary hyperparathyroidism will ensue with a consequent increase in plasma level of PTH. This condition is commonly encountered in patients with chronic kidney disease especially with advanced stages and has been proposed to be correlated with certain complications commonly seen in such patients including cardiovascular diseases and renal osteodystrophy. For this reason, the prognostic value of PTH in patients with chronic kidney disease has received great emphasis.

2. Secondary hyperparathyroidism

Next to vitamin D deficiency, chronic kidney disease is known to be the second most common cause of secondary hyperparathyroidism. The prevalence of secondary hyperparathyroidism in such patients is strongly correlated with the stage of CKD. In other words, plasma PTH concentration is negatively correlated with glomerular filtration rate (GFR) in patients with CKD. Around 80% of patients with GFR of less than 20 mL/min/1.73 m^2 has an increased level of PTH [1]. At the early stages of CKD, the major stimulus of the parathyroid glands is the hyperphosphatemia caused by impaired renal excretion of phosphorus in addition to impaired activation of vitamin D. Prolonged exposure to hyperphosphatemia and development of hypocalcemia in concurrence with high levels of fibroblast growth factor (FGF)-23 will lead to overproduction of PTH where hyperplasia of the parathyroid tissue ensues with persistent exposure to these metabolic abnormalities [2]. FGF-23 plays an indirect role in regulating the synthesis and secretion of PTH for being involved in regulating renal excretion of phosphate in addition to renal production of activated vitamin D. Furthermore, increasing studies suggest a direct role of FGF-23 in suppressing PTH synthesis and secretion through a direct action on the parathyroid glands. This inhibitory effect is significantly impaired in patients with CKD [3]. Persistent overstimulation of parathyroid glands is associated with hyperplasia that is categorized into 4 types which are diffuse hyperplasia, diffuse and multinodular hyperplasia, multinodular hyperplasia, and simple nodular hyperplasia [4]. Various clinical consequences are characteristic of secondary hyperparathyroidism including bone and soft tissue, skin and cardiovascular manifestations. Extraosseous calcification is the main pathophysiology of many clinical manifestations as it involves arterial walls, cutaneous tissue, viscera and even cornea and conjunctiva. This calcification is also correlated with the increased mortality rate in patients with CKD as it might involve myocardium and endocardium and the arterial walls of the aorta and coronary arteries leading to significant ventricular dysfunction, heart failure, ischemia, arrhythmia and death [5]. This might explain the increasing emphasis by many authors on serial measurement of plasma PTH in patients with CKD as a part of management.

3. Parathyroid hormone

Parathyroid hormone is an amino acid hormone composed of 84 amino acids, synthesized in the parathyroid glands. It is initially synthesized as pre-pro-PTH with 115 amino acids that is converted into pro-PTH with 90 amino acids. The latter will be cleaved to form the active form of PTH. The response of parathyroid glands to hypocalcemia by secreting PTH is so powerful. This response occurs within seconds of hypocalcemia in an attempt to rapidly restore normal plasma calcium levels. In addition to de novo synthesis, PTH is stored in secretory granules within the parathyroid glands and both represent the sources of circulatory PTH. The stored PTH within the parathyroid glands explains the rapid release of PTH from the parathyroid glands in response to short term hypocalcemia while prolonged hypocalcemia stimulates synthesis and release of PTH by parathyroid glands [6]. The estimated half-life of PTH is only a few minutes after which it is rapidly eliminated from circulation by the liver and kidneys [7]. The direct action of PTH involves three main organs; bone, kidneys and small intestine. In respect of its effect on the bones, PTH plays a vital role in releasing calcium to the circulation indirectly through the activation of osteoclasts (bone resorption). This action is preceded by stimulating the differentiation of osteoblasts into osteoclasts. This effect of PTH on the bones has a great impact on the rapid correction of plasma calcium levels in short-term hypocalcemia. On the kidneys, PTH has multiple functions that are essential in maintaining plasma calcium levels. At the distal convoluted tubules and collecting ducts, PTH mediates the reabsorption of calcium that has not been reabsorbed at the proximal convoluted tubules. Furthermore, PTH enhances the elimination of phosphate by decreasing the rate of its reabsorption, an action that is indirectly participating in maintaining plasma calcium as less phosphate will be available to bind with plasma free calcium [8]. Another vital action of PTH on the kidney includes increasing the production of 1 alpha-hydroxylase in the proximal convoluted tubules. The final step of activation of vitamin D is catalyzed by this enzyme. This active form of vitamin D mediates the absorption of calcium by the intestine in both transcellular and paracellular pathways in addition to its role in preventing loss of calcium in urine by enhancing its reabsorption at the distal convoluted tubules [9]. Currently, PTH is measured using the second generation intact PTH assay which has the ability to detect various PTH fragments including full-length (1–84) PTH and long C-PTH fragments, primarily (7–84) PTH, although the differences in the effects of each fragment on various systems in the body are not clear yet [10].

4. Correlation of parathyroid hormone and certain medical conditions

The higher incidence of certain medical conditions that have been observed in patients with high levels of plasma PTH has raised the suspicion of a possible role of PTH in the development of these conditions whether directly or indirectly. The indirect action is represented by alteration of plasma calcium concentration in form of hypercalcemia or hypocalcemia with their known impact on the function of various body organs. The direct action of PTH is related to its ability to bind to a G-protein-coupled receptor (PTH1R) leading to its activation with subsequent downstream activation of adenylyl cyclase and protein kinase A pathway or phospholipase C/protein kinase C (PKC) pathway according to the target organ [11]. This sequence of events when occurs within the cardiomyocytes will trigger further steps that end with excessive growth of cardiomyocytes and left ventricular hypertrophy [12]. The prevalence of hypertension in patients with primary hyperparathyroidism is extremely high reaching 40–60% [13]. Various mechanisms have been suggested for this correlation such as activation protein kinase C, exaggerated cardiovascular reactivity to norepinephrine, amplified effects of the renin-angiotensin system and many others [14]. Furthermore, altered glucose metabolism and even diabetes have been reported in patients with high plasma PTH concentration due to inhibition of insulin signaling in adipocytes via adenylate cyclase and phosphorylation of IRS-1 on serine 307 [15]. Approximately 8–22% of patients with primary hyperparathyroidism have type 2 diabetes mellitus and around 1% of patients with type 2 diabetes have primary hyperparathyroidism [16]. Although rare, acute pancreatitis has been as an initial presentation in patients with high plasma PTH levels due to a parathyroid gland tumor [17]. PTH has been correlated with metabolic syndrome, hyperlipidemia and coronary artery disease by many clinical studies [18–20]. For all this evidence, estimation of plasma PTH concentration should be a central step in the plan of management of many critical and highly prevalent medical conditions.

5. Plasma PTH level in patients with CKD

CKD is defined as progressive irreversible loss of renal function with associated metabolic disorders secondary to parenchymal renal damage. The severity of metabolic disorders associated with CKD is inversely related to glomerular filtration rate (GFR). Secondary hyperparathyroidism is an expected finding in patients with CKD caused by various factors related to impaired renal function including hyperphosphatemia, hypocalcemia and low levels of activated vitamin D. Consequently, persistently high levels of plasma PTH is an expected finding in patients with CKD. An important question is to determine whether this increase in PTH is considered an adaptive response or an exaggerated one. This has influenced some authors to calculate GFR-specific cutoff for PTH to differentiate between the two possibilities before considering PTH as a prognostic marker [21]. The major impact of PTH in patients with CKD is on bone metabolism and it is considered as the main cause for the development of mineral bone disease in such patients. Plasma PTH increases progressively at the early stages of CKD in an attempt to correct hyperphosphatemia. It is estimated that around 20% of patients with CKD have increased PTH concentration at GFR of more than 60 mL/min/1.73 m^2 compared to 40% at Stage 3, 70% at Stage 4, and > 80% at Stage 5 [22]. The role of PTH as a prognostic marker in patients with CKD was thoroughly studied and numerous studies have confirmed this role. For this reason, the National Kidney Foundation's Kidney disease outcomes Quality Initiative (KDOQI) clinical practice guidelines recommend routine measurement of plasma PTH early in the course of CKD [23]. Furthermore, Kidney Disease Improving Global Outcomes (KDIGO) has recommended that PTH should be routinely checked in patients with CKD at stages 3–5 [24].

5.1 Prognostic value of plasma PTH in patients with CKD

Many deleterious consequences are known to be correlated with increased plasma PTH in patients with CKD including progressive deterioration of renal function, anemia, impaired response to erythropoietin in addition to many other medical conditions. The cardiovascular mortality rate is significantly increased even before reaching stage 5 [25]. This explains PTH being considered as a uremic toxin due to its extraskeletal effects [26]. These effects are thought to be related to the increase in intracellular calcium in various cells, apart from smooth muscle cells, secondary to a decreased efflux and an increased influx of calcium into the cells. Since the leading cause of death in patients with CKD is cardiovascular disease, the correlation between plasma PTH and cardiovascular disease in such patients has been reviewed thoroughly and it is worthy to start with this correlation when discussing the prognostic value of PTH in patients with CKD.

5.2 PTH and cardiovascular disease

It is well known that patients with end-stage kidney disease have an increased risk of cardiovascular disease of 5–10 times higher than the general population making it a challenge because it represents the major cause of death in such group of patients knowing that CKD represents a relatively highly prevalent medical condition where, in the USA, more than 50% of patients aged over 65 years have CKD [27]. The correlation between plasma PTH and the risk of all-cause and cardiovascular mortality has been confirmed when this risk was greatly reduced by parathyroidectomy. Various mechanisms have been implicated to explain this correlation. For example, cardiac sympathetic overdrive in addition to impaired vagal control in late stages of CKD was associated with arrhythmia which is responsible for sudden cardiac death in patients with CKD especially those on hemodialysis [28] which represents two-thirds of the total cardiovascular mortality in this group of patients. Altered cardiac autonomic modulation presented as decreased heart rate variability (obtained using 24-h Holter examinations) has been reported in patients with CKD and has been considered as a mortality risk predictor [29] where high plasma PTH was significantly correlated with decreased heart rate variability in patients with CKD on hemodialysis. Interaction between PTH and phosphorus, vitamin D and FGF-23 has been implicated in the development of this correlation [30]. Left ventricular cardiomyopathy represents the most frequent cardiac abnormality in patients on dialysis where left ventricular hypertrophy (LVH) is present in 60–75% of patients before initiating dialysis and up to 90% have LVH after dialysis. Although the pathophysiology of CKD-related cardiomyopathy is multifactorial, high plasma PTH is considered to have the main role in the development of this condition although other factors have been recently implicated including FGF-23 [31]. The findings during the histopathological study of post-mortem cardiac tissue were an increase in diameter of cardiomyocytes, reduced density of capillary length and an increase in interstitial volume [32]. Furthermore, diffused interstitial fibrosis has been observed in cardiac tissue in advanced cases of CKD and has been partially linked to PTH among other factors [33]. Many clues are present about the vascular effect of PTH and its association with hypertension and stroke. In respect to the correlation of PTH and hypertension in patients with CKD, elevated blood pressure has been normalized in patients on hemodialysis when treated with parathyroidectomy [34, 35] or etelcalcetide [36]. On the other hand, certain studies have revealed a strong predictive value of PTH and ischemic stroke especially in the presence of 25 (OH)D. The latter seems to have the highest predictive value even when compared to hypertension and high PTH [37]. In addition, increasing attempts are present to determine a reliable biomarker that can detect patients with CKD who have a higher risk of cardiovascular mortality. So, in addition to the conventional biomarkers, PTH and phosphorus, newer ones such as FGF23, Klotho, and sclerostin might have a slightly better prognostic value. In respect to FGF23, it is thought to represent a biomarker of the bone-heart axis as it might be a link between bone metabolism and cardiac function [38]. A higher concentration of circulating FGF-23 has been correlated with an increased risk of cardiovascular disease in patients with CKD where LVH and heart failure were significantly higher [39]. Various clinical studies have suggested that a progressive increase of circulating FGF-23 in patients with CKD was associated with a significant increase in all-cause mortality [40, 41]. Similarly, soluble klotho, co-receptor for FGF-23, has been investigated for its correlation with morbidity and mortality in patients with CKD. It has been shown that the prevalence of cardiovascular events was much higher in patients with low klotho concentration irrespective of other predictors of cardiovascular disease in patients with CKD [42]. Furthermore, low serum klotho has been associated with higher all-cause mortality even after adjustment of other confounders [43].

It is worthy to mention that even in the presence of normal renal function, high plasma PTH levels are associated with increased risk of coronary artery disease and heart failure [44] but this correlation requires further studies as certain authors have not confirmed it.

5.3 PTH and anemia

Anemia is a highly prevalent finding in patients with CKD and is considered as a sign of poor prognosis as it is associated with increased cardiovascular disease, hospitalization and mortality. Up to 100% of patients with stage 5 KCD have anemia. It is of a different pathophysiological basis although erythropoietin deficiency is the most recognized underlying cause. Other causes include resistance to erythropoietin, bone marrow fibrosis and shortened life span of red blood cells [45]. Secondary hyperparathyroidism and the associating high PTH level have been linked to these suggested causes of anemia. Bone marrow fibrosis has been detected in both primary and secondary hyperparathyroidism with consequent anemia which is significantly improved after parathyroidectomy making the correlation of bone marrow fibrosis and secondary hyperparathyroidism highly suggestive [46, 47]. Fortunately, bone marrow fibrosis has been reversed after parathyroidectomy. The direct inhibitory effect of PTH on erythropoietin synthesis has been confirmed by many authors when plasma concentration of erythropoietin increased significantly after parathyroidectomy reaching to 10-folds higher than its preoperative concentration within 2 weeks or even less; the molecular pathophysiology of this inhibitory effect is not yet known [48, 49]. Shortened lifespan of red blood cells has been observed in patients with CKD as a cause of anemia and it was linked to the high plasma PTH due to its role in increasing median osmotic fragility of red blood cells with consequent anemia [50]. Cinacalcet hydrochloride, a calcimimetic drug, which is used as a medical treatment of secondary hyperparathyroidism has been associated with improvement in hemoglobin level and necessitating fewer doses of erythropoiesis-stimulating agents to correct anemia [51, 52]. Similarly, patients with CKD and secondary hyperparathyroidism treated with the active form of vitamin D (calcitriol) have shown a similar response to that of cinacalcet with improved hemoglobin level and less doses of erythropoietin required to control anemia [53].

5.4 PTH and mortality rate in patients with CKD

The triad of altered calcium and phosphorus metabolism and high plasma PTH level represents one of the major challenges during the management of patients with CKD due to their adjuvant harmful consequences on various body tissues and their correlation to the high mortality rate commonly observed in patients with CKD with the leading cause being the cardiovascular disease. These disorders of metabolism are associated with accelerated vascular calcification involving various arteries including coronary arteries. Both hypercalcemia and hyperphosphatemia that are present in patients with prolonged secondary hyperparathyroidism seen in patients with CKD are associated with medial calcification. Furthermore, skin and soft tissue necrosis and ulceration, known as uremic arteriolopathy or calciphylaxis, is an uncommon serious complication of secondary hyperparathyroidism and has an eight-fold increase in mortality [54]. Many studies have suggested PTH as an independent risk factor for renal death in patients with CKD whether on renal replacement therapy or not [55, 56]. The severity of increase of PTH prior to hemodialysis has been shown to predict more difficulty in decreasing PTH afterwards [57]. It is of great importance to notify that a low or even normal concentration of PTH is thought to be associated with poor prognosis as well. KDIGO recommend plasma concentration of PTH to be 2–9 times the upper normal limit [57]. A gradual decrease of PTH to the target level has been associated with a significant decrease in mortality rate. Patients with concomitant high plasma concentrations of PTH and phosphorus have shown a higher risk of mortality [58]. The residual renal function seems to be a determinant factor for the risk of mortality in patients with high plasma PTH. Many clinicians are attracted to normalize PTH using various modalities including vitamin D, phosphate binders and calcimimetics but their benefit in reducing the mortality rate is questioned depending on various clinical studies that failed to confirm an association between the improvement in biochemical and hematological parameters and reduction of the risk of mortality rate suggesting more precautions for the use of these modalities in an attempt to reduce the risk of renal death [59]. In contrast, a recent meta-analysis study enrolling around 25000 patients has suggested a significant beneficial effect of parathyroidectomy in reducing mortality rate explained by controlling blood pressure and improvement of left ventricular hypertrophy [60].

All these findings highlight the importance of plasma PTH in the management of patients with CKD making it a cornerstone in the course of the illness as it affects various tissues and organs in the body in addition to its confirmed correlation with the risk of mortality in such patients.

Author details

Raid D. Hashim
Al-Rasheed University College, Baghdad, Iraq

*Address all correspondence to: vsdasd9@gmail.com

References

[1] Van Der Plas W, Noltes M, Van Ginhoven T, Kruijff S. Secondary and tertiary hyperparathyroidism: a narrative review. Scandinavian Journal of Surgery. 2020; 109(4): 271-278.

[2] Komaba H, Fukagawa M. FGF23–parathyroid interaction: implications in chronic kidney disease. Kidney International. 2010;77(4):292-298.

[3] Mace ML, Gravesen E, Nordholm A, Olgaard K, Lewin E. Fibroblast growth factor (FGF) 23 regulates the plasma levels of parathyroid hormone in vivo through the FGF receptor in normocalcemia, but not in hypo calcemia. Calcified tissue international. 2018;102(1):85-92.

[4] Xu D, Yin Y, Hou L, Dai W. Surgical management of secondary hyperparathyroidism: how to effectively reduce recurrence at the time of primary surgery. Journal of endocrinological investigation. 2016;39(5):509-514.

[5] Wilkieson TJ, Rahman MO, Gangji AS, Voss M, Ingram AJ, Ranganath N, et al. Coronary artery calcification, cardiovascular events, and death: a prospective cohort study of incident patients on hemodialysis. Canadian Journal of Kidney Health and Disease. 2015;2:29.

[6] Tinawi M. Disorders of calcium metabolism: hypocalcemia and hypercalcemia. Cureus. 2021;13(1).

[7] Chen H, Han X, Cui Y, Ye Y, Purrunsing Y, Wang N. Parathyroid Hormone Fragments: New Targets for the Diagnosis and Treatment of Chronic Kidney Disease-Mineral and Bone Disorder. BioMed Research International. 2018;2018:9619253-.

[8] Prasad N, Bhadauria D. Renal phosphate handling: Physiology. Indian journal of endocrinology and metabolism. 2013;17(4):620.

[9] Christakos S, Lieben L, Masuyama R, Carmeliet G. Vitamin D endocrine system and the intestine. BoneKEy Reports. 2014;3.

[10] Huimin C, Ying C, Changying X, Xiaoming Z, Yan Z, Qingting W, et al. Effects of Parathyroidectomy on Plasma iPTH and (1-84) PTH Levels in Patients with Stage 5 Chronic Kidney Disease. Hormone and Metabolic Research. 2018;50(10):761-767.

[11] Schlüter KD. PTH and PTHrP: Similar Structures but Different Functions. News in Physiological Sciences. 1999;14:243-249.

[12] Brown SJ, Ruppe MD, Tabatabai LS. The Parathyroid Gland and Heart Disease. Methodist DeBakey Cardiovascular Journal. 2017;13(2): 49-54.

[13] Pepe J, Cipriani C, Sonato C, Raimo O, Biamonte F, Minisola S. Cardiovascular manifestations of primary hyperparathyroidism: a narrative review. European Journal of Endocrinology. 2017;177(6):R297-R308.

[14] Fisher SB, Perrier ND. Primary hyperparathyroidism and hypertension. Gland Surgery. 2020;9(1):142-149.

[15] Chang E, Donkin SS, Teegarden D. Parathyroid hormone suppresses insulin signaling in adipocytes. Molecular and Cellular Endocrinology. 2009;307(1-2): 77-82.

[16] Ghigo E, Porta M. Diabetes secondary to endocrine and pancreatic disorders: Karger Medical and Scientific Publishers; 2014.

[17] Gao Y, Yu C, Xiang F, Xie M, Fang L. Acute pancreatitis as an initial

manifestation of parathyroid carcinoma: A case report and literature review. Medicine. 2017;96(44):e8420.

[18] Mendoza-Zubieta V, Gonzalez-Villaseñor GA, Vargas-Ortega G, Gonzalez B, Ramirez-Renteria C, Mercado M, et al. High prevalence of metabolic syndrome in a mestizo group of adult patients with primary hyperparathyroidism (PHPT). BMC Endocrine Disorders. 2015;15:16.

[19] Tassone F, Gianotti L, Baffoni C, Cesario F, Magro G, Pellegrino M, et al. Prevalence and characteristics of metabolic syndrome in primary hyperparathyroidism. Journal of Endocrinological Investigation. 2012;35(9):841-846.

[20] Han D, Trooskin S, Wang X. Prevalence of cardiovascular risk factors in male and female patients with primary hyperparathyroidism. Journal of Endocrinological Investigation. 2012;35(6):548-552.

[21] Canney M, Djurdjev O, Tang M, Zierold C, Blocki F, Wolf M, et al. GFR-Specific versus GFR-Agnostic Cutoffs for Parathyroid Hormone and Fibroblast Growth Factor-23 in Advanced Chronic Kidney Disease. American Journal of Nephrology. 2019;50(2):105-114.

[22] Wei Y, Lin J, Yang F, Li X, Hou Y, Lu R, et al. Risk factors associated with secondary hyperparathyroidism in patients with chronic kidney disease. Experimental and Therapeutic Medicine. 2016;12(2):1206-1212.

[23] Kramer H. The national kidney foundation's kidney disease outcomes quality initiative (KDOQI) grant initiative: moving clinical practice forward. American Journal of Kidney Diseases. 2010;55(3):411-414.

[24] Kidney Disease: Improving Global Outcomes CKDMBDUWG. KDIGO 2017 Clinical Practice Guideline Update for the Diagnosis, Evaluation, Prevention, and Treatment of Chronic Kidney Disease-Mineral and Bone Disorder (CKD-MBD). Kidney International Supplements (2011). 2017;7(1):1-59.

[25] Tentori F, Wang M, Bieber BA, Karaboyas A, Li Y, Jacobson SH, et al. Recent changes in therapeutic approaches and association with outcomes among patients with secondary hyperparathyroidism on chronic hemodialysis: the DOPPS study. Clinical Journal of the American Society of Nephrology. 2015;10(1):98-109.

[26] Rodriguez M, Lorenzo V. Parathyroid hormone, a uremic toxin. Seminars in Dialysis. 2009;22(4): 363-368.

[27] Saran R, Robinson B, Abbott KC, Agodoa LYC, Bragg-Gresham J, Balkrishnan R, et al. US Renal Data System 2018 Annual Data Report: Epidemiology of Kidney Disease in the United States. American Journal of Kidney Diseases. 2019;73(3 Suppl 1):A7-a8.

[28] Clyne N, Hellberg M, Kouidi E, Deligiannis A, Höglund P. Relationship between declining glomerular filtration rate and measures of cardiac and vascular autonomic neuropathy. Nephrology (Carlton). 2016;21(12):1047-1055.

[29] Chandra P, Sands RL, Gillespie BW, Levin NW, Kotanko P, Kiser M, et al. Predictors of heart rate variability and its prognostic significance in chronic kidney disease. Nephrology Dialysis Transplantation. 2012;27(2):700-709.

[30] Cunningham J, Locatelli F, Rodriguez M. Secondary hyperparathyroidism: pathogenesis, disease progression, and therapeutic options. Clinical Journal of the

American Society of Nephrology. 2011;6(4):913-921.

[31] Hruska KA, Seifert M, Sugatani T. Pathophysiology of the chronic kidney disease-mineral bone disorder. Current Opinion in Nephrology and Hypertension. 2015;24(4):303-309.

[32] Amann K, Breitbach M, Ritz E, Mall G. Myocyte/capillary mismatch in the heart of uremic patients. Clinical Journal of the American Society of Nephrology. 1998;9(6):1018-1022.

[33] de Albuquerque Suassuna PG, Sanders-Pinheiro H, de Paula RB. Uremic Cardiomyopathy: A New Piece in the Chronic Kidney Disease-Mineral and Bone Disorder Puzzle. Frontiers of Medicine (Lausanne). 2018;5:206.

[34] Shih CJ, Tarng DC, Yang WC, Yang CY. Parathyroidectomy reduces intradialytic hypotension in hemodialysis patients with secondary hyperparathyroidism. Kidney and Blood Pressure Research. 2013;37(4-5): 323-331.

[35] Sofronie AC, Kooij I, Bursot C, Santagati G, Coindre J-P, Piccoli GB. Full normalization of severe hypertension after parathyroidectomy – a case report and systematic review. BMC Nephrology. 2018;19(1):112.

[36] Simeoni M, Perna AF, Fuiano G. Secondary Hyperparathyroidism and Hypertension: An Intriguing Couple. Journal of Clinical Medicine. 2020;9(3):629.

[37] Çelik G, Doğan A, Dener Ş, Öztürk Ş, Kulaksızoğlu S, Ekmekçi H. Parathyroid Hormone Levels in the Prediction of Ischemic Stroke Risk. Disease Markers. 2017;2017:4343171-.

[38] Stöhr R, Schuh A, Heine GH, Brandenburg V. FGF23 in Cardiovascular Disease: Innocent Bystander or Active Mediator? Frontiers in Endocrinology (Lausanne). 2018;9:351.

[39] Scialla JJ, Wolf M. Roles of phosphate and fibroblast growth factor 23 in cardiovascular disease. Nature Reviews Nephrology. 2014;10(5): 268-278.

[40] Bouma-de Krijger A, de Roij van Zuijdewijn CLM, Nubé MJ, Grooteman MPC, Vervloet MG, Group tCS. Change in FGF23 concentration over time and its association with all-cause mortality in patients treated with haemodialysis or haemodiafiltration. Clinical Kidney Journal. 2020;14(3):891-897.

[41] Xue C, Yang B, Zhou C, Dai B, Liu Y, Mao Z, et al. Fibroblast Growth Factor 23 Predicts All-Cause Mortality in a Dose-Response Fashion in Pre-Dialysis Patients with Chronic Kidney Disease. American Journal of Nephrology. 2017;45(2):149-159.

[42] Memmos E, Sarafidis P, Pateinakis P, Tsiantoulas A, Faitatzidou D, Giamalis P, et al. Soluble Klotho is associated with mortality and cardiovascular events in hemodialysis. BMC Nephrology. 2019;20(1):217.

[43] Otani-Takei N, Masuda T, Akimoto T, Honma S, Watanabe Y, Shiizaki K, et al. Association between Serum Soluble Klotho Levels and Mortality in Chronic Hemodialysis Patients. International Journal of Endocrinology. 2015;2015:406269-.

[44] Kestenbaum B, Katz R, de Boer I, Hoofnagle A, Sarnak MJ, Shlipak MG, et al. Vitamin D, parathyroid hormone, and cardiovascular events among older adults. Journal of the American College of Cardiology. 2011;58(14):1433-1441.

[45] Tanaka M, Komaba H, Fukagawa M. Emerging association between parathyroid hormone and anemia in hemodialysis patients. Therapeutic

Apheresis and Dialysis. 2018;22(3): 242-245.

[46] Rao DS, Shih M-S, Mohini R. Effect of Serum Parathyroid Hormone and Bone Marrow Fibrosis on the Response to Erythropoietin in Uremia. New England Journal of Medicine. 1993;328(3):171-175.

[47] Brancaccio D. Hyperparathyroidism and Anemia in Uremic Subjects: A Combined Therapeutic Approach. Journal of the American Society of Nephrology. 2004;15(90010):21S-214.

[48] Ureña P, Eckardt K-U, Sarfati E, Zingraff J, Zins B, Roullet JB, et al. Serum erythropoietin and erythropoiesis in primary and secondary hyperparathyroidism: effect of parathyroidectomy. Nephron. 1991;59(3):384-393.

[49] Washio M, Iseki K, Onoyama K, Oh Y, Nakamoto M, Fujimi S, et al. Elevation of serum erythropoietin after subtotal parathyroidectomy in chronic haemodialysis patients. Nephrology Dialysis Transplantation. 1992;7(2):121-124.

[50] Shaaban HSM, Khamis SSA, Mohamed YSY, Kasem HES, Omar TA. Parathyroid Hormone as a Marker for the Red Cell Fragility in Different Stages of Chronic Kidney Disease. Open Journal of Nephrology. 2021;11(01):123.

[51] Mpio I, Boumendjel N, Karaaslan H, Arkouche W, Lenz A, Cardozo C, et al. [Secondary hyperparathyroidism and anemia. Effects of a calcimimetic on the control of anemia in chronic hemodialysed patients. Pilot Study]. Néphrologie & Thérapeutique. 2011;7(4):229-236.

[52] Tanaka M, Yoshida K, Fukuma S, Ito K, Matsushita K, Fukagawa M, et al. Effects of Secondary Hyperparathyroidism Treatment on Improvement in Anemia: Results from the MBD-5D Study. PLoS ONE. 2016;11(10):e0164865.

[53] Aucella F, Scalzulli RP, Gatta G, Vigilante M, Carella AM, Stallone C. Calcitriol increases burst-forming unit-erythroid proliferation in chronic renal failure. A synergistic effect with r-HuEpo. Nephron Clinical Practice. 2003;95(4):c121-c127.

[54] Mazhar AR, Johnson RJ, Gillen D, Stivelman JC, Ryan MJ, Davis CL, et al. Risk factors and mortality associated with calciphylaxis in end-stage renal disease. Kidney international. 2001;60(1):324-332.

[55] Borrelli S, Chiodini P, De Nicola L, Minutolo R, Provenzano M, Garofalo C, et al. Prognosis and determinants of serum PTH changes over time in 1-5 CKD stage patients followed in tertiary care. PLoS ONE. 2018;13(8):e0202417.

[56] Rodriguez M, Lorenzo V, editors. Progress in uremic toxin research: parathyroid hormone, a uremic toxin. Seminars in dialysis; 2009: Wiley Online Library.

[57] Tabibzadeh N, Karaboyas A, Robinson BM, Csomor PA, Spiegel DM, Evenepoel P, et al. The risk of medically uncontrolled secondary hyperparathyroidism depends on parathyroid hormone levels at haemodialysis initiation. Nephrology Dialysis Transplantation. 2020;36(1): 160-169.

[58] Wang M, Obi Y, Streja E, Rhee CM, Lau WL, Chen J, et al. Association of parameters of mineral bone disorder with mortality in patients on hemodialysis according to level of residual kidney function. Clinical Journal of the American Society of Nephrology. 2017;12(7):1118-1127.

[59] Goldsmith D, Covic A, Vervloet M, Cozzolino M, Nistor I, group CKD-MBDw, et al. Should patients with CKD

stage 5D and biochemical evidence of secondary hyperparathyroidism be prescribed calcimimetic therapy? An ERA-EDTA position statement. Nephrology Dialysis Transplantation. 2015;30(5):698-700.

[60] Apetrii M, Goldsmith D, Nistor I, Siriopol D, Voroneanu L, Scripcariu D, et al. Impact of surgical parathyroidectomy on chronic kidney disease-mineral and bone disorder (CKD-MBD)–A systematic review and meta-analysis. PLoS One. 2017;12(11): e0187025.

Chapter 9

Cardiorenal Syndrome in Patients on Renal Replacement Therapy

Evgeny Shutov and Natalia Filatova

Abstract

In this chapter authors discusses cardiorenal relationships in patients with renal replacement therapy (RRT) which are considered as a separate type of cardiorenal syndrome (CRS). Frequency and severity of CRS in patients on dialysis are correlated with quantity of years of the dialysis treatment; depend on quality of dialysis regimen and level of residual renal function. RRT-associated cardiac pathology are including left ventricular hypertrophy, ischemic cardiomyopathy, congestive heart failure, coronary atherosclerosis and calcinosis, severe arrhythmias. The article analyzes role of malnutrition and dialysis-induced cachexia, bio-incompatibility of dialysis membranes, oxidative stress and inflammation, arterio-venous fistula, decrease of residual renal function in the development of dialysis-induced CRS. The review examines the mechanisms of progressive myocardial ischemia induced by dialysis: myocardial stunning, hemodialysis-induced hypotension, uremic small vessel disease. Prevention of dialysis-induced CRS includes a choice of the optimal RRT method (peritoneal dialysis or hemodialysis), control of dialysis regimen, residual renal function, biocompatibility of membrane, inflammatory markers, body mass index, serum level albumin, phosphate, calcium, parathyroid hormone, fibroblast growth factor-23. Electrocardiogram, ultrasonic monitoring and coronarography reveals indications for conservative cardioprotective therapy and angioplasty interventions, including coronary artery bypass surgery and cardiac pacemaker implantation, in patients with dialysis-induced CRS.

Keywords: cardiorenal syndrome, hemodialysis, peritoneal dialysis, residual renal function, oxidative stress, malnutrition

1. Introduction

Cardiorenal syndrome (CRS) refers to the "vicious circle" of interrelated damage of the heart and kidneys, in which dysfunction of one organ complicates the dysfunction of the other, with gradual development of the cardiorenal decompensation.

C. Ronco distinguished 5 clinical types of CRS [1]:

Type 1: Acute worsening of heart function leading to kidney injury and/or dysfunction.

Type 2: Chronic abnormalities in heart function leading to kidney injury or dysfunction. This subtype refers to a more chronic state of kidney disease complicating chronic heart disease, the so-called chronic kidney disease (CKD).

IntechOpen

Type 3: Acute worsening of kidney function leading to heart injury and/or dysfunction (acute heart failure).
Type 4: Chronic kidney disease causing cardiac overload, leading to progressive chronic cardiac dysfunction.
Type 5: Systemic condition (e.g., sepsis, vasculitis) leading to simultaneous injury and/or dysfunction of heart and kidney.

We can see the interplay of decreased glomerular filtration rate and impaired cardiac contractile function early in chronic kidney disease (CKD) worsening as renal failure increases. However, the existing classification of CRS does not consider the population of patients on renal replacement therapy (RRT), where the effect of dialysis treatment itself engages additional mechanisms of pathogenesis of cardiac pathology. Thus, the progression of cardiac dysfunction with decreasing ejection fraction reduces the effectiveness of hemodialysis (HD), while reducing the intensity of dialysis regimen and gradual loss of residual renal function speeds up the atherosclerosis and cardiomyopathy progression.

Thus, one can consider the cardiorenal relationships in patients on RRT, reflecting progression and myocardial damage in dialysis patients, as a separate type of CRS where the renal component implies end stage renal disease (ESRD) with complicating metabolic and endocrine disorders, complete loss of residual renal function, and dialysis therapy.

The features of cardiac dysfunction in patients on RRT include its widespread prevalence and severity [2]. The incidence of left ventricular myocardial hypertrophy (LVH) increases with increasing stage of CKD, reaching 90% in stages 4–5 [3]. Prevalence and severity of cardiac pathology, both coronary and non-coronary, increases rapidly in the dialysis stage of renal failure, correlating with dialysis experience. In 75–80% of patients with CKD stage 5D, secondary cardiomyopathy develops predisposing to congestive heart failure (CHF), acute coronary syndrome, or complex rhythm and conduction abnormalities. In patients on RRT, progressive atherosclerosis is associated with activation of inflammatory reactions and high frequency of protein-energy malnutrition (PEM) [4]. Thus, PEM is diagnosed in 20–50% of patients with pre-dialysis stages of CKD, increasing to 50–80% in patients on regular HD and permanent PD.

The cardiac function in patients on RRT deteriorates progressively under several pathogenetic mechanisms. These include bio-incompatibility of dialysis membranes and solutions, ineffective dialysis, PEM, dialysis hypotension, rapid decline and subsequent complete loss of residual renal function, vascular calcification, excessive shunt from arterio-venous hemodialysis fistula (AVF).

2. Bio-incompatibility of dialysis membranes, activation of oxidative stress, and inflammation

CKD in RRT is characterized by higher level of uremia and the impact of dialysis procedure itself. Despite the successes of modern hemodialysis therapy, the problem of hemodialysis membranes' bio-incompatibility is still unresolved. A key inducer of blood cell activation is dialyzer membrane material, along with the endotoxin contamination of dialysis solutions. Membrane contact with blood causes pro-inflammatory and pro-oxidant stress, thrombosis, and release of oxidative stress biomarkers, inflammatory and anti-inflammatory cytokines (IFN-γ, TNF-α, IL -1β, IL-4, IL-6, IL-10, IL-12, and IL-18), and acute phase proteins (C-reactive protein, fibrinogen) [5]. Other consequences of bio-incompatibility are complement [6] and platelet activation [7].

The oxidative events induced by extracorporeal treatment are thought to affect the concomitant pathology. Chronic inflammation, besides cardiovascular dysfunction, contributes to worsening renal anemia by reducing sensitivity to the erythropoietin-stimulating agent and shortening the life span of red blood cells [8, 9]. Also, blood leukocyte activation, oxidative stress, and mechanical factors damage the red blood cells. Leukocytes in contact with bio-incompatible dialysis membranes re-activate. The resultant leukopeniais considered a major cause of defective cellular immune response in patients on hemodialysis (HD) [10, 11]. Changes in lymphocyte phenotype (from Th1 to Th2) cause this response and excessive synthesis of pro-inflammatory cytokines [5]. Bio-incompatible membranes release pyrogens and active inflammatory mediators (histamine and bradykinin). These contribute to fever and hemodialysis-induced hypotension [12]. The latter is a key factor in residual renal function reducing in patients on regular HD [13].

Dialysate composition for peritoneal dialysis (PD) can also cause oxidative stress and inflammation [14, 15]. High concentrations of glucose and lactate, and low pH or hyperosmolality of dialysate for PD contribute to excessive production of reactive oxygen species and accumulation of oxidative damage products in the peritoneum, increasing calcification and fibrosis. The relationship between the preserved residual renal function and oxidative stress has been shown to correlate with cardiovascular risk and survival in patients on PD [14]. Given the longer preservation of residual renal function in patients on PD treatment, this method can be considered more favorable for patients with cardiovascular diseases (CVD). Also, several studies have shown a higher accumulation of oxidants and depletion of antioxidant reserves in patients on HD compared with those on PD [15, 16].

The accumulation of oxidative stress products is the highest in patients with ESRD. Peroxidizing agents oxidize unsaturated lipids [17–19] and endogenous pro-oxidants damage plasma proteins with the formation of glycation products [20–22]. Small reactive carbonyls and larger posttranslational uremic-modified proteins form many inflammatory mediators, reflecting uremic toxicity that is little dependent on the method of dialysis therapy [23]. However, all modern diffusion, convective, or mixed methods do not remove medium- and high-molecular-weight dissolved substances modified by reactive oxygen species (ROS) and reactive carbonyls effectively from blood [24–26].

Oxidative stress plays a key role in the development of cardiac dysfunction in patients on RRT. In patients with ESRD, the balance between nitric oxide (NO) and ROS is shifted toward the latter by increasing ROS production and decreasing NO availability [27]. Pro-inflammatory cytokines such as IL-1β, IL-6, TNF-α can stimulate renin synthesis and norepinephrine secretion [28, 29]. IL-6 induces AT-1 receptors and angiotensin II-mediated ROS production in cultured rat smooth muscle cells, supporting the link between inflammation, renin-angiotensin-aldosterone system (RAAS) activation, and oxidative stress [30]. Volume overload on RRT and venous stasis are additional sources of inflammatory mediators [31, 32]. Because of intravascular overload, the vascular endothelium may be a major source of cytokine production in response to biomechanical stress [33]. Thus, the above data confirms the potential role of circulating cellular precursors of ROS and/or local agonists of ROS synthesis in the development of CRS in dialysis patients.

C. Vida et al. have shown in dialysis patients the activation of peripheral blood polymorphonuclear and mononuclear leukocytes, which leads to excess production of oxidative compounds such as reactive oxygen species, and it is this process that plays the leading role [34].

The imbalance between the RAAS, sympathetic nervous system, and inflammation speeds up the CRS formation in dialysis patients. To prevent and slow the cardiac pathology in HD treatment, highly purified dialysis solutions and synthetic dialysis membranes are being developed to reduce the risk of oxidative stress and other manifestations caused by low biocompatibility of membranes. For example, dialysis membranes made of regenerated cellulose that interact with the β-D-glucose hydroxyl groups of blood components cause activation of the complement system and leukopenia. To improve the biocompatibility of these membranes, hydroxyl groups are modified chemically by acetylation to produce triacetate cellulose or addition of D-α-tocopherol polyethylene glycol-1000 succinate chains, an esterified form of α-tocopherol. HD and PD in CKD permanently excrete antioxidants through the membranes. To normalize their blood levels and suppress ROS generation in patients on HD, vitamins C, E, and glutathione are supplemented orally [27].

3. Protein and energy deficiency and dialysis cachexia

PEM should be noted among the factors influencing the progression of cardiovascular pathology and the formation of CRS in patients on dialysis [35, 36]. Progressive blood pressure instability with LVH and diastolic dysfunction, acidosis, coronary atherosclerosis, as well as increasing hypoalbuminemia and severe anemia early lead to ineffective HD and loss of residual renal function. These exacerbate hyperhydration with overload and ischemia of myocardial muscle, oxidative stress, and heart chamber dilatation.

The causes of PEM in dialysis patients include protein hypercatabolism with decreased synthesis of albumin and essential amino acids and their subsequent losses (more on PD), L-carnitine deficiency, anorexia with depression, and chronic inflammation with hyperproduction of pro-inflammatory cytokines [37]. Uremic hyperparathyroidism with deficiency of anabolic hormones (insulin, erythropoietin) plays an important role in the PEM development. Progression of PEM is fixed by monitoring of anthropometry (BMI, shoulder muscle circumference, and triceps skinfold), levels of albumin, lymphocytes, TNF-α, transferrin, and CRP.

In the advanced stage of dialysis CRS, PEM progresses to MIA-syndrome (Malnutrtion, Inflammation, Atherosclerosis). This is manifested by ischemic cardiomyopathy provoking arrhythmias, stenotic atherosclerosis with diffuse calcification of arteries and heart valves, and treatment-resistant anemia and hypoalbuminemia [38].

Dialysis cachexia in MIA syndrome is formed in BMI under 15 kg/m^2 with hypoalbuminemia (<30 g/l). Clinically it manifests by severe cardiovascular, endocrine, and immune disorders [39]. It is characteristic of the late stage of CRS, when dialysis cachexia is aggravated by cachexia of chronic heart failure (CHF). The formed CHF aggravates PEM because of acidosis with additional hypercatabolism, oxidative stress, impaired absorption syndrome and hypoalbuminemia, and polypragmasia. These patients have poorly controlled hypertension with recurrent intra-dialysis hypotension, ischemic cardiomyopathy with arrhythmias, widespread coronary atherosclerosis and calcinosis, severe hyperparathyroidism, and encephalopathy. There is a high risk of dementia and infection with outcome in bacterial sepsis. Successful treatment of anorexia, hypoalbuminemia, infectious complications, and encephalopathy is possible only with a comprehensive correction of depression, immunodeficiency (anti-cytokines, antibiotics), anemia, amino acid and L-carnitine deficiency, tube (parenteral) feeding, and infusion of proteins. In severe cachexia, kidney transplantation is effective.

4. Influence of residual kidney function reduction on progression of cardiovascular pathology in patients on RRT

Preservation of residual kidney function in dialysis patients improves their survival and prognosis. For example, Dutch joint NECOSAD study [40] in 740 patients on HD showed an increase in residual kidney function (Kt/V by 1 unit) associated with a 66% reduction in the relative risk of death. Prospective analysis by W. Van der Wal et al., which included 1800 dialysis patients (1191 patients were on HD and 609 on PD), found a 1.5-fold death risk increase after loss of residual renal function compared to patients with preserved residual renal function [41]. Y. Obi et al. found that higher and more stable residual renal function (GFR) was associated with better patient survival one year after initiation of regular HD. Mortality related inversely with residual renal function measured by urea clearance and daily urine output [42]. In several other multicenter studies [43, 44] residual function has been an independent predictor of survival in patients on PD. The Canadian-American Study (CANUSA) [45] showed on 601 patients on PD that residual renal function rather than peritoneal creatinine clearance and peritoneal ultrafiltration (UF) correlate with patient survival. A study of residual renal function in PD patients showed a 36% reduction in the relative risk of death with an increase in daily urine output by 250 mL.

Preservation of residual renal function provides better control of hyperhydration, dyselectrolytemia, inflammatory activity, and clearance of protein-bound low molecular weight toxins and medium-molecular-weight molecules. Even a small amount of residual function reduces the level of plasma dissolved uremic toxins and β_2-microglobulin [46–48].

The residual renal function allows to reduce cardiac mortality and progression of cardiovascular disease in dialysis patients primarily through better hydration control. Both on regular and continuous PD, CKD patients with uncorrected hyperhydration are at high risk of developing cardiovascular complications: volume/sodium-dependent hypertension, left ventricular hypertrophy, arrhythmias, and congestive heart failure [49–51]. The expansion of intravascular volume leads to elongation of myocardial cells, and eccentric or asymmetrical left ventricular remodeling [52].

In patients on intermittent HD, UF causes post-ischemic impairment of myocardial contractile function (myocardial stunning) even in the absence of angiographically significant coronary disease [53]. Recurrent UF-induced ischemia provokes chronic left ventricular dysfunction, a cause of CHF progression in patients on HD [54]. Preserved residual renal function in patients on regular PD allows to reduce UF volumes during dialysis session, thus reducing risk of recurrent myocardial ischemia or systolic pressure drop during the session (hemodialysis-induced hypotension) [54–57]. In patients on PD, maintenance of residual renal function and significant diuresis attenuates the damaging effects of dextrose on the peritoneal membrane and reduces hyperglycemia and the risk of obesity and diabetes.

The residual renal function not only increases survival but also improves hormonal, mineral-bone, and nutritional disorders and the quality of life in patients on HD and PD, as confirmed by the CHOICE study [58]. Higher quality of life in patients with diuresis over 250 ml per day is also associated with a less restriction in diet and fluid intake, and better nutritional status [59] and control of hyperphosphatemia, renal osteodystrophy, and anemia. The latter depend on a renal synthesis of erythropoietin and active forms of vitamin D_3 in kidneys [60, 61]. Several data have shown an association between the preserved residual renal function and decreased production of inflammatory markers: C-reactive protein and interleukin-6 [62, 63].

5. Ultrafiltration, hemodialysis-induced hypotension and metabolic acidosis

In patients with end stage CKD, fluid removal is achieved by extracorporeal UF with HD or intracorporeal UF with continuous PD. Unlike intermittent HD, continuous PD is not associated with “stunned” myocardium, which largely explains the slower progression of CHF in patients treated with PD [64]. However, clinical studies showed contradictory results on the benefits of PD. V. Panday et al. found in a retrospective analysis of 139 patients with CKD stage 5 and concomitant CHF no difference in two-year mortality, cardiac outcomes, and hospitalization rates between patients on PD and HD [65]. In a study using the Taiwan National Database with over 35,000 patients, I. Wang et al. showed lower survival of ESRD patients and comorbid CHF on the PD treatment [66]. However, the findings could be related to difficulties in hydration management on PD, complete loss of residual renal function, and/or shortcomings and limitations of the analysis performed. In a registry analysis in Lombardy, F. Locatelli et al. found no significant difference in the magnitude of cardiovascular risk in the groups treated with HD compared to that on PD [67]. Recent studies based on the Taiwan National Registry (2016), which included over 45,000 patients with end stage CKD, showed the 29% higher risk of cardiovascular disease in patients treated with HD compared to those treated with PD [68].

The development of intradialysis hypotension on regular HD is caused by uremic polyneuropathy and CHF, when, in response to dialysis UF, the vascular bed fills inadequately slowly, causing hypovolemia and hypotension. Dialysis CRS with hypotension is often complicated by thrombosis of vascular access, resulting in rapid formation of underdialysis syndrome with hypercatabolism. Blood loss and sinus tachycardia combined with hemodialysis-induced hypotension significantly increase the risk of acute coronary syndrome and cerebrovascular accident (CVA). Patients with diabetic nephropathy often develop severe hemodialysis-induced hypotension refractory to conservative therapy. The hypotension can provoke target organ ischemia. Vasopressors and alpha-adrenergic agonists are not safe in treating hemodialysis-induced hypotension. Controlled UF with “dry weight” monitoring by bio-impedance, transfer to PD, or daily (nighttime) HD are recommended.

Metabolic acidosis is common in patientswith ESRD because of a decreased ability to excrete acids and reduced renal synthesis of bicarbonate. It leads to malnutrition, inflammation, bone disease disorders, and even a higher death risk [69]. Significant acid–base variations during dialysis may play an important role in CVD development in HD patients. One study [70] has shown an association between low serum bicarbonate concentrations and cardiovascular disease in patients on dialysis. It is important to avoid large variations in serum bicarbonate levels in dialysis patients because these variations can increase CVD.

6. Stenotic atherosclerosis

MIA syndrome is characterized by rapid stenosing of the major arteries by the progressing atherosclerosis combined with calcinosis. Frequent complications are ischemic kidney disease with uncontrolled renin-dependent hypertension, stenotic atherosclerosis of cerebral arteries with the risk of CVA, ischemic occlusive enteropathy with malabsorption syndrome aggravating PEM and anemia.

In dialysis CRS with the expanded PEM, coronary heart disease (CHD) is typical with unstable angina and elevated blood CRP correlating with LDL levels [71, 72]. Hyperparathyroidism is associated with progressive coronary artery calcification, increasing atherosclerosis [73, 74]. Stenosis of the proximal coronary artery is typical, which causes high mortality in patients on dialysis [75]. Early diagnosis of myocardial infarction in dialysis CRS is difficult because of confounding uremic polyneuropathy, dyselectrolitemia, myocardial calcification, and coronary calcinosis. Coronarography in 60% of patients with CKD stage 5 admitted for regular HD treatment in Japan reveals low-symptomatic stenosis of one coronary artery and of several coronary arteries (multivessel disease) in some patients.

To prevent acute coronary syndrome, risk factors should be addressed in HD: hemodialysis-induced hypotension, sinus tachycardia, blood loss, and anemia. ACE inhibitors reduce the cardiac mortality [76]. Nitrates and beta-blockers are tolerated worse in dialysis CRS because of hemodynamic instability.

Hemodialysis-induced myocardial ischemiamight regress with the use of beta-blockers, which have substantially improved survival in patients with acute coronary syndromes and heart failure. In dialysis patients, carvedilol significantly improved cardiovascular mortality, LV function, and LV morphology. Dialysis patients treated with carvedilol had a 50% lower mortality rate than patients receiving placebo [77, 78]. The efficacy of statins on regular HD has not been proven conclusively, and the incidence of side effects is higher than in the early stages of CKD [79].

Current guidelines by KDIGO recommend not starting lipid-lowering therapy in dialysis patients. These recommendations are based on clinical trials which failed to show that statin therapy is beneficial in reducing cardiovascular mortality indialysis patients, in contrast to the general population [80]. High-density lipoprotein cholesterol (HDL-C) from HD patients compared to healthy controls has been much less effective in cholesterol efflux and regulation of inflammation [81]. HDL-C from HD patients promotes endothelial dysfunction via accumulation of symmetric dimethylarginine (SDMA), which is associated with increased all-cause and cardiovascular mortality [82].

Erythropoietin drugs cannot fully realize their cardioprotective effect because of more frequent side effects of the high doses. Survival rate after acute myocardial infarction is extremely low at conservative therapy of CHD on hemodialysis (by the end of the 1st year, 41%, after 2 years, 27%, after 3 years, 10%). This causes intolerance of uremic myocardium to ischemia with small coronary artery remodeling (uremic small vessel disease) and myocardial stunning on HD. In coronary angioplasty in patients with dialysis-related CRS, the acute postoperative mortality is over 3.5 times higher than the statistical average, and the long-term survival rate after stenting is significantly higher than in conservative therapy [83].

7. Progressive CHF with low cardiac output

CHF in patients on HD is manifested by worsening chronic hypervolemia, causing both circuits decompensation and a significant decrease in ejection fraction preventing effective HD, and development of critical progressive hyponatremia with a high risk of cerebral edema. The 3-year survival rate of patients with CHF on regular HD does not exceed 20%, and sudden cardiac death is most frequent fatality in this group of patients on HD [84].

The rate of sudden cardiac death is 59 deaths in 1000 patient-years in the CKD stage 5D population, whereas it is 1 death in 1000 patient-years in the general population [85]. Patients on dialysis have a high incidence of coronary heart disease, but the rate of sudden cardiac death is disproportionately high compared with the incidence of coronary heart disease in these patients. Even a complete revascularization reduce the risk of sudden cardiac death only in part [86]. Dialysis, especially HD, is a risk factor for sudden cardiac death, providing the highest risk within the first 12 hours after dialysis and after a long dialysis-free interval [87]. Potential mechanisms include volume and sudden electrolyte shifts after dialysis, volume overload, and electrolyte disturbance.

These outcomes largely depend not on the severity of CHD, but on the value of the corrected QT-interval and QT dispersion and are caused by complex rhythm disturbances in dialysis malnutrition (hypercatabolism, acidosis, imbalance of potassium, sodium and calcium in dialysis solution, and hypomagnesemia) [88]. Cardioprotectors, antiarrhythmics, and vasopressors provide only short-term effect; myocardial reperfusion, artificial pacemaker, implanted cardioverter-defibrillator are more effective [84, 88].

PD may be the method of choice in the treatment of patients with CHF, providing effective UF and sodium excretion in the required volumes, especially when using icodextrin solution. In patients with CRS and severe ascites, PD can reduce intra-abdominal pressure. PD in patients with CHF has several advantages: continuous "mild" UF with minimal impact on hemodynamics and reduction of volume overload symptoms; weight reduction and correction of hypervolemia; increase in left ventricular ejection fraction; sodium "sieving" effect and better control of hypernatremia; removal of acute phase proteins, medium-molecular-weight molecules, abscence of pro-inflammatory activation of cytokines; reduction of intraabdominal pressure and improved quality of life in patients with severe ascites; and better control of serum potassium level with the possibility of using aldosterone receptor blockers and ACE inhibitors. Heart transplantation should be used in refractory cases, sometimes in combination with the kidney transplantation.

8. Vascular calcification

Hyperparathyroidism, frequent in RRT patients, is prognostically unfavorable [89]. Elevation of serum fibroblast growth factor-23 (FGF-23) with the development of resistance to it precedes Mineral Bone Disease (MBD). Elevated FGF23 levels were independently associated with LVH.FGF23 caused LVH via FGF receptor-dependent activation of the calcineurin-nuclear factor of activated T-cells signaling pathway [90]. Klotho deficiency and FGF23 elevation are associated with poor outcomes and complications in dialysispatients. Klotho deficiency cause vascular calcification, cardiac fibrosis, and cardiac hypertrophy in patients with CKD [91].

Hyperphosphatemia and parathyroid hormone elevation increase with increasing stage of CKD and correlate with cardiac mortality [92]. This is largely because of vascular calcification, especially pronounced in dialysis patients, which is associated with the use of solutions for PD and HD with increased calcium content.

Vascular calcification (VC) is defined as vascular deposition of calcium-phosphate mineral complexes. Traditionally, two forms of calcification are pointed out: 1) intimal calcification in proximity to lipid deposits, clinically relevant in obstructive arterial disease and 2) medial calcification with differentiation of smooth muscle cells into osteoblast-like cells is akin to bone formation, related to several genes as BMP2, Msh Homeobox 2, and gene of alkaline phosphatase [93].

Medial calcification is common in dialysis patients with CKD.VC has a clearrelationship with atherosclerotic vascular disease [94]. Calcification of arterial vessels leads to arterial stiffness, contributes to increased pulse wave velocity, increased cardiac afterload, and thus heart failure [95]. Arterial stiffness is an independent predictor of cardiovascular mortality [96]. Arterial stiffness and medial calcification intensify each other, to create a vicious cycle [97]. Heart valve calcification occurs in stage 5 CKD in up to 88–99% of patients, increasing from 40% of patients in CKD stage 3 [98].

Calcinosis of heart valves leads to the formation of acquired heart valvular disease (aggravating CHF) and increases the risk of infective endocarditis. The extent of vascular calcifications in CKD herald a poor prognosis [99]. Resulting hemodynamic alterations induce left ventricular hypertrophy associated with a decrease in coronary perfusion [100].

In dialysis CRS, active vitamin D metabolites are contraindicated because of the risk of soft tissue calcification (including skin calcification with sepsis). Calcium-free phosphate binders are advisable: sevelamer, lanthanum carbonate [101]. Sevelamer corrects hyperphosphatemia and decreases mortality in dialysis patients by 1.5 times, slowing coronary calcification, reducing blood levels of atherogenic lipids, FGF-23, and pro-inflammatory cytokines [102]. Iron-containing phosphate binders effectively lower blood phosphate levels, but are often complicated by diarrhea and nutritional disorders exacerbation in PEM [103]. Total parathyroidectomy in patients with dialysis cachexia is effective in MBD and CHF progression but carries a risk of acute postoperative complications [104]. An alternative to parathyroidectomy is administration of calcimimetics. Prolonged-release cinalcet reduces the need for parathyroidectomy, slows arterial and cardiac valve calcification, and reduces cardiovascular mortality [105, 106].

9. Immunodeficiency

In dialysis-associated CRS, infection is severe, both induced by thrombosis of sclerosed AVF or not associated with vascular access. Pneumonia risk factors in dialysis CRS with malnutrition include immune deficiency with activation of opportunistic infections and Staphylococcus carrying in the nasopharynx, CHF with chronic hyperhydration and hypoxia of lung tissue, hydrothorax, hyperparathyroidism with lung tissue calcification, obstructive night apnea syndrome, and epoetin-resistant anemia.

Pathogens of acute pneumonia on dialysis include staphylococcus, opportunistic bacteria (*E. Coli*, Haemophylis influenzae, Klebsiella, Pseudomonas, Listeria, Legionella), and pathogenic fungi (Aspergillus, Candida, Cryptococcus, Mucormyces). In dialysis CRS, the mortality is extremely high from pneumonia caused by the association of influenza virus with *Staphylococcus aureus* [107] or superinfection with pneumocysts in MIA syndrome patients infected with cytomegalovirus. At the advanced stage of CRS in diabetic patients, purulent complications of obliterating atherosclerosis of lower limb arteries and diabetic foot typically cause high mortality from gangrene and sepsis. Risk factors for infectious endocarditis in dialysis CRS are vascular access infection, calcinosis of valves in severe hyperparathyroidism, their myxomatous degeneration, thrombotic deposits, or severe anemia [108].

Antibiotic therapy is carried out after removal of the infected fistula with the formation of a new AVF or with transfer to PD [109]. Treatment with broad-spectrum antibiotics should be started immediately and corrected by the blood culture results. Antibiotic therapy is ineffective in CHF, recurrent thromboembolism, fungal endocarditis, tricuspid or pulmonary artery valves lesions (frequent in HD patients). In these cases, surgery is necessary to replace the affected valve [108].

10. Epoetin-resistant anemia

Anemia in CKD patients induces eccentric LVH and exacerbates myocardial ischemia, increasing cardiovascular mortality in dialysis CRS [110, 111]. Erythropoietin drugs improve the quality of life of dialysis patients. However, the mortality-reducing effect of erythropoietin in dialysis CRS has not been proven, and the most effective and safe target Hb level is not established. The currently recommended target Hb level of 10–12 g/dL does not stimulate sufficiently neoangiogenesis and endothelial stem cells activity.

Resistant anemia often develops within MIA syndrome (under the influence of chronic inflammation, acidosis, iron malabsorption, vit. B12 and folic acid deficiency), as well as because of ineffective HD syndrome and hyperparathyroidism, requiring the unusually high doses of erythropoietin. Since this therapy is often complicated by poorly controlled hypertension and thrombosis, combined antihypertensive therapy, complete correction of iron deficiency, vit. B12 and metabolic acidosis, and control of the coagulation system are indicated [112]. Intensification of HD regimen, correction of hyperparathyroidism, influence on chronic inflammation syndrome (anti-cytokine drugs, etc.) are of great importance for overcoming resistance to epoetin. At critically low hemoglobin, blood transfusions can be used.

Recently, a new group of drugs has been proposed to treat anemia, the so called hypoxia-inducible factor-prolyl hydroxylase inhibitors (HIF-PHIs). HIF-PHIs promote erythropoiesis primarily through increased endogenous EPO production and modulation of iron metabolism. The results of phase 2 and 3 clinical trials have shown their advantages, such as decreased hepcidin levels, better iron utilization and thus less need for iron, the ability to influence the background of inflammation without increasing the dose [113]. These drugs will probably find their use in patients with epoetin-resistant anemia associated with both inflammation and iron metabolism disorders.

11. Impact of arterio-venous hemodialysis fistula

In dialysis patients, one can assume the relationship between CHF and recent AVF formation in slight reduction of cardiac output, absence of pulmonary hypertension and other causes of heart failure progression (severe CHD, cardiomyopathy).

After AVF formation, peripheral vascular resistance decreases rapidly, leading to compensatory increase of cardiac output and possibly to acute CHF decompensation. Because of the increase of blood inflow to the heart, the diastolic size of the left ventricleand pulmonary pressure increase [114]. Subsequently, progressing myocardial hypertrophy and dilatation of heart cavities cause diastolic LV dysfunction and CHF development [115]. Pulmonary hypertension, found in 40–50% of patients on HD [116], joins soon after AVF formation and is associated with the size of arterio-venous shunt [117]. The inadequate pulmonary vasodilation in response to the AVF-induced increase in blood flow rate is thought to be caused by decreased NO synthesis in the endothelium or accumulation of uremic NO inhibitors, such as asymmetric dimethyl arginine [118].

In all patients on regular HD, AVF with a large shunt should be considered as a factor aggravating the CHD and CHF development. Normalization of blood flow in AVF can lead to delay in cardiovascular pathology progression. In peripheral bypass syndrome, blood flow and perfusion in the limb distal to the fistula reduce dramatically because of shunt redistribution of blood flow. Less known is coronary bypass syndrome, where left-sided AVF, bypassing the left internal thoracic artery, reduces coronary blood flow, which can lead to myocardial ischemia, especially during the HD session [119].

After the AVF formation, the blood volume increases to maintain a higher cardiac output and can be complicated by severe (refractory) hypertension. In several "preload (end-diastolic pressure)-dependent" dialysis patients, poorly controlled dialysis-induced hypotension accompanies inter-dialysis hypertension in the first 15–20 min of HD even with moderate volumes of UF. Among other complications, fistula infection with outcome in progressing CHF and thromboembolic syndrome provokes prognostically unfavorable bacterial endocarditis.

Thus, AVF, being essentially an iatrogenic vascular anomaly formed to treat HD, can contribute to cardiac mortality. The negative effect of AVF on cardiovascular mortality is directly proportional to blood flow in the fistula and severity of initial cardiovascular pathology. Thus, AVF should not be used in patients with LV ejection fraction <40% and significant pulmonary hypertension. Therefore, the AVF formation should be preceded by cardiac assessment (ECG and Echo-CG monitoring) involving a consultation with a cardiologist.

AVF formation should be planned 2–3 months before the expected start of HD. It is unwise to form AVF a year or more before the start of HD and at Hb levels >12 g/dL because of high risk of fistula thrombosis. Blood flow in the fistula should be targeted at 400–600 ml/min; for blood flow over 800 ml/min, surgical reduction of arterio-venous blood shunt is reasonable. Ultrasonography, venography, and arteriography (fistulography) are used to monitor AVF.

In patients with refractory CHF, CHD with unstable angina, coronary or peripheral bypass syndrome, or severe pulmonary hypertension, AVF ligation with transfer to CAPD is indicated. In endocarditis after removal of infected AVF is recommended temporary transfer of a patient with HD to CAPD or low-flow dialysis, increasing the effectiveness of antibiotic therapy, followed by prosthetic heart valves insertion. PD can be used also for the period of standard AVF formation and maturation instead of AVF with excessive shunt.

12. Conclusion

Further study is important of cardiorenal relationships in patients on RRT with the isolation of a separate "dialysis-related" type of CRS reflecting the progression of cardiac dysfunction during dialysis treatment. To analyze the features of dialysis CRS, a comprehensive approach should be developed for its treatment and prevention.

Author details

Evgeny Shutov[1,2]* and Natalia Filatova[2]

1 Botkin Clinical City Hospital, Moscow, Russian Federation

2 Russian Medical Academy of Continuous Professional Education, Moscow, Russian Federation

*Address all correspondence to: shutov_e_v@mail.ru

References

[1] Ronco C, McCullough P, Anker SD, et al. Cardio-renal syndromes: report from the consensus conference of the acute dialysis quality initiative. Eur Heart J. 2010; 31(6):703-711. doi:10.1093/ eurheartj/ ehp507

[2] Vanholder R, Massy Z, Argiles A, et al. Chronic kidney disease as a cause of cardiovascular morbidity and mortality. Nephrol Dial Transplant. 2005; 20(6):1048-1056. doi:10.1093/ ndt/gfh813

[3] Zoccalli C. Cardiorenal risk as a new frontier of nephrology: research needs and areas for intervention. Nephrol Dial Transplant. 2002; 17 Suppl 11:50-54. doi:10.1093/ndt/17.suppl_11.50

[4] London G, Marchais S, Guerin A, et al. Inflammation, arteriosclerosis, and cardiovascular therapy in hemodialysis patients. Kidney Int Suppl. 2003; 84:S88-S93. doi:10.1046/j. 1523-1755.63.s84.25.x

[5] Libetta C, Sepe V, Esposito P, Galli F, Dal Canton A. Oxidative stress and inflammation: implications in uremia and hemodialysis. Clin Biochem. 2011; 44(14-15):1189-1198. doi:10.1016/j. clinbiochem.2011.06.988

[6] Mares J, Richtrova P, Hricinova A, et al. Proteomic profiling of blood-dialyzer interactome reveals involvement of lectin complement pathway in hemodialysis-induced inflammatory response. Proteomics Clin Appl. 2010; 4(10-11):829-838. doi:10.1002/prca.201000031

[7] Brunini T, Mendes-Ribeiro A, Ellory J, Mann G. Platelet nitric oxide synthesis in uremia and malnutrition: a role for L-arginine supplementation in vascular protection? Cardiovasc Res. 2007; 73(2):359-367. doi:10.1016/j. cardiores.2006.09.019

[8] Locatelli F, Del Vecchio L, Pozzoni P, Andrulli S. Dialysis adequacy and response to erythropoiesis-stimulating agents: what is the evidence base? Semin Nephrol. 2006; 26(4):269-274. doi:10.1016/j.semnephrol.2006.05.002

[9] Elliott J, Mishler D, Agarwal R. Hyporesponsiveness to erythropoietin: causes and management. Adv Chronic Kidney Dis. 2009; 16(2):94-100. doi:10.1053/j.ackd.2008.12.004

[10] Van der Steen A. Research on dialyzers with improved biocompatibility. Clin Nephrol. 1986; 26 Suppl 1:S39-S42. PMID:3829466

[11] Rousseau Y, Carreno MP, Poignet JL, Kazatchkine MD, Haeffner-Cavaillon N. Dissociation between complement activation, integrin expression and neutropenia during hemodialysis. Biomaterials. 1999; 20(20):1959-1967. doi:10.1016/s0142-9612(99)00101-5

[12] Del Vecchio L, Locatelli F, Carini M. What we know about oxidative stress in patients with chronic kidney disease on dialysis – clinical effects, potential treatment, and prevention. Semin Dial. 2011; 24(1):56-64. doi:10.1111/j. 1525-139X.2010.00819.x

[13] Jansen M, Hart A, Korevaar J, et al; NECOSAD Study Group. Predictors of the rate of decline of residual renal function in incident dialysis patients. Kidney Int. 2002; 62(3):1046-1053. doi:10.1046/j.1523-1755.2002.00505.x

[14] Liakopoulos V, Roumeliotis S, Gorny X,Eleftheriadis T, Mertens PR. Oxidative stress in patients undergoing peritoneal dialysis: a current review of the literature. Oxid Med Cell Longev. 2017; 2017:3494867. doi:10.1155/ 2017/3494867

[15] Roumeliotis S, Eleftheriadis T, Liakopoulos V. Is oxidative stress an

issue in peritoneal dialysis? Semin Dial. 2019; 32(5):463-466. doi:10.1111/sdi.12818

[16] Krata N, Zagożdżon R, Foroncewicz B, Mucha K. Oxidative stress in kidney diseases: the cause or the consequence? Arch Immunol Ther Exp (Warsz). 2018; 66(3):211-220. doi:10.1007/s00005-017-0496-0

[17] Ikizler T, Morrow J, Roberts L, et al. Plasma F2-isoprostane levels are elevated in chronic hemodialysis patients. Clin Nephrol. 2002; 58(3):190-197. doi:10.5414/cnp58190

[18] Ferraro B, Galli F, Frei B, et al. Peroxynitrite-induced oxidation of plasma lipids is enhanced in stable hemodialysis patients. Kidney Int. 2003; 63(6):2207-2213. doi:10.1046/j.1523-1755.2003.00008.x

[19] Muller C, Eisenbrand G, Gradinger M, et al. Effects of hemodialysis, dialyser type and iron infusion on oxidative stress in uremic patients. Free Radic Res. 2004; 38(10):1093-1100. doi:10.1080/10715760400011452

[20] Galli F, Benedetti S, Floridi A, Canestrari F, Piroddi M. Glycoxidation and inflammatory markers in patients on treatment with PMMA-based protein-leaking dialyzers. Kidney Int. 2005; 67(2):750-759. doi:10.1111/j.1523-1755.2005.67138.x

[21] Piroddi M, Palmese A, Pilolli F, et al. Plasma nitroproteome of kidney disease patients. Amino Acids. 2011; 40(2):653-667. doi:10.1007/s00726-010-0693-1

[22] Thornalley P, Rabbani N. Protein damage in diabetes and uremia – identifying hotspots of proteome damage where minimal modification is amplified to marked pathophysiological effect. Free Radic Res. 2011; 45(1):89-100. doi:10.3109/10715762.2010.534162

[23] Vanholder R, Baurmeister U, Brunet P, et al. A bench to bedside view of uremic toxins. J Am Soc Nephrol. 2008; 19(5):863-870. doi:10.1681/ASN.2007121377

[24] Vanholder R, Schepers E, Meert N, Lameire N. What is uremia? Retention versus oxidation. Blood Purif. 2006; 24(1):33-38. doi:10.1159/000089434

[25] De Smet R, Dhondt A, Eloot S, et al. Effect of the super-flux cellulose triacetate dialyser membrane on the removal of non-protein-bound and protein-bound uraemic solutes. Nephrol Dial Transplant. 2007; 22(7):2006-2012. doi:10.1093/ndt/gfm065

[26] Thomas G, Jaber B. Convective therapies for removal of middle molecular weight uremic toxins in end-stage renal disease: a review of the evidence. Semin Dial. 2009; 22(6):610-614. doi:10.1111/j.1525-139X.2009.00665.x

[27] Galli F, Piroddi M, Annetti C, et al. Oxidative stress and reactive oxygen species. Contrib Nephrol. 2005; 149: 240-260. doi:10.1159/000085686

[28] Sanchez-Lozada LG, Tapia E, Johnson RJ, Rodríguez-Iturbe B, Herrera-Acosta J. Glomerular hemodynamic changes associated with arteriolar lesions and tubulointerstitial inflammation. Kidney Int Suppl. 2003; 86:S9-14. doi:10.1046/j.1523-1755.64.s86.3.x

[29] Niijima A, Hori T, Aou S, Oomura Y. The effects of interleukin-1β on the activity of adrenal, splenic and renal sympathetic nerves in the rat. J Auton Nerv Syst. 1991; 36(3):183-192. doi:10.1016/0165-1838(91)90042-2

[30] Wassmann S, Stumpf M, Strehlow K, et al. Interleukin-6 induces oxidative stress and endothelial dysfunction by overexpression of the angiotensin II type 1 receptor. Circ Res.

2004; 94(4):534-541. doi:10.1161/01. RES.0000115557.25127.8D

[31] Tsutamoto T, Hisanaga T, Wada A, et al. Interleukin-6 spillover in the peripheral circulation increases with the severity of heart failure, and the high plasma level of interleukin-6 is an important prognostic predictor in patients with congestive heart failure. J Am Coll Cardiol. 1998; 31(2):391-398. doi:10.1016/s0735-1097(97)00494-4

[32] Anker SD, Egerer KR, Volk HD, et al. Elevated soluble CD14 receptors and altered cytokines in chronic heart failure. Am J Cardiol. 1997; 79:1426-1430. doi:10.1016/s0002-9149(97) 00159-8

[33] Kawai M, Naruse K, Komatsu S, et al. Mechanical stress-dependent secretion of interleukin 6 by endothelial cells after portal vein embolization: clinical and experimental studies. J Hepatol. 2002; 37(2):240-246. doi:10.1016/s0168-8278(02)00171-x

[34] Vida C, Oliva C, Yuste C, et al. Oxidative stress in patients with advanced ckd and renal replacement therapy: the key role of peripheral blood leukocytes. Antioxidants (Basel). 2021; 10(7):1155. doi:10.3390/antiox10071155

[35] Gama-Axelsson T, Heimburger D, Stevinkel P, et al. Serum albumin as predictor of nutritional status in patients with ESRD. Clin J Am Soc Nephrol. 2012; 7(9):1446-1453. doi:10.2215/CJN.10251011

[36] Carrero JJ, Avesani CM. Pros and cons of body mass index as a nutritional and risk assessment tool in dialysis patients. Semin Dial. 2015; 28(1): 48-58. doi:10.1111/sdi.12287

[37] Kovesdy CP. Malnutrition in dialysis patients - the need for intervention despite uncertain benefits. Semin Dial. 2016; 29(1):28-34. doi:10.1111/sdi.12410

[38] Kalantar-Zadeh K, Ikizler TA, Block G, Avram MM, Kopple JD. Malnutrition-Inflammation complex syndrome in dialysis patients: causes and consequences. Am J Kidney Dis. 2003; 42(5):864-881. doi:10.1016/j. ajkd.2003.07.016

[39] De Roij van Zuijdewijn CL, ter Wee PM, Chapdelaine I, et al. A comparison of 8 nutrition-related tests to predict mortality in haemodialysis patients. J Ren Nutr. 2015; 25(5):412-419. doi:10.1053/j.jrn.2015.02.005

[40] Termorshuizen F, Dekker FW, van Manen JG, et al; NECOSAD Study Group. Relative contribution of residual renal function and different measures of adequacy to survival in hemodialysis patients: an analysis of the Netherlands cooperative study on the adequacy of dialysis (NECOSAD)-2. J Am Soc Nephrol. 2004; 15(4):1061-1070. doi:10.1097/01.asn.0000117976. 29592.93

[41] van der Wal WM, Noordzij M, Dekker FW, et al. Full loss of residual renal function causes higher mortality in dialysis patients; findings from a marginal structural model. Nephrol Dial Transplant. 2011; 26(9):2978-2983. doi:10.1093/ndt/gfq856

[42] Obi Y, Streja E, Rhee C, et al. Incremental hemodialysis, residual kidney function, and mortality risk in incident dialysis patients: a cohort study. Am J Kidney Dis. 2016; 68(2):256-265. doi:10.1053/j.ajkd.2016.01.008

[43] Diaz-Buxo JA, Lowrie EG, Lew NL, et al. Associates of mortality among peritoneal dialysis patients with special reference to peritoneal transport rates and solute clearance. Am J Kidney Dis. 1999; 33(3):523-534. doi:10.1016/ s0272-6386(99)70190-3

[44] Rocco M, Soucie JM, Pastan S, McClellan WM. Peritoneal dialysis adequacy and risk of death. Kidney Int.

2000; 58(1):446-457. doi:10.1046/j.1523-1755.2000.00184.x

[45] Bargman JM, Thorpe KE, Churchill DN. Relative contribution of residual renal function and peritoneal clearance to adequacy of dialysis: a reanalysis of the CANUSA study. J Am Soc Nephrol. 2001; 12(10):2158-2162. doi:10.1681/ASN.V12102158

[46] Kabanda A, Jadoul M, Pochet JM, et al. Determinants of the serum concentrations of low molecular weight proteins in patients on maintenance hemodialysis. Kidney Int. 1994; 45(6):1689-1696. doi:10.1038/ki.1994.221

[47] Stompór T., Sułowicz W., Anyszek T. et al. Dialysis adequacy, residual renal function and serum concentrations of selected low molecular weight proteins in patients undergoing continuous ambulatory peritoneal dialysis. Med Sci Monit. 2003; 9(11):CR500-CR504. PMID:14586277

[48] Delaney MP, Stevens PE, Al Hasani M, et al. Relationship of serum cystatin C to peritoneal and renal clearance measures in peritoneal dialysis: a cross-sectional study. Am J Kidney Dis. 2008; 51(2):278-284. doi:10.1053/j.ajkd.2007.08.018

[49] Gunal AI, Kirciman E, Guler M, Yavuzkir M, Celiker H. Should the preservation of residual renal function cost volume overload and its consequence left ventricular hypertrophy in new hemodialysis patients? Ren Fail. 2004; 26(4):405-409. doi:10.1081/jdi-120039825

[50] Voroneanu L, Cusai C, Hogas S, et al. The relationship between chronic volume overload and elevated blood pressure in hemodialysis patients: use of bioimpedance provides a different perspective from echocardiography and biomarker methodologies. Int Urol Nephrol. 2010; 42(3):789-797. doi:10.1007/s11255-010-9767-y

[51] Hassan K, Hassan S, Anwar S, et al. Predictors of left ventricular hypertrophy and their cutoffs in peritoneal dialysis patients. Int Heart J. 2015; 56(2):186-191. doi:10.1536/ihj.14-246

[52] Di Lullo L, Gorini A, Russo D, Santoboni A, Ronco C. Left ventricular hypertrophy in chronic kidney disease patients: from pathophysiology to treatment. Cardiorenal Med. 2015; 5(4):254-266. doi:10.1159/000435838

[53] McIntyre CW, Burton JO, Selby NM, et al. Hemodialysis-induced cardiac dysfunction is associated with an acute reduction in global and segmental myocardial blood flow. Clin J Am Soc Nephrol. 2008; 3(1):19-26. doi:10.2215/CJN.03170707

[54] Burton JO, Jefferies HJ, Selby NM, McIntyre CW. Hemodialysis-induced repetitive myocardial injury results in global and segmental reduction in systolic cardiac function. Clin J Am Soc Nephrol. 2009; 4(12):1925-1931. doi:10.2215/CJN.04470709

[55] Burton JO, Jefferies HJ, Selby NM, McIntyre CW. Hemodialysis-induced cardiac injury: determinants and associated outcomes. Clin J Am Soc Nephrol. 2009; 4(5): 914-920. doi:10.2215/CJN.03900808

[56] Dorairajan S, Chockalingam A, Misra M. Myocardial stunning in hemodialysis: what is the overall message? Hemodial Int. 2010; 14(4):447-450. doi:10.1111/j.1542-4758.2010.00495.x

[57] McIntyre CW. Haemodialysis-induced myocardial stunning in chronic kidney disease – a new aspect of cardiovascular disease. Blood Purif. 2010; 29(2):105-110. doi:10.1159/000245634

[58] Shafi T, Jaar BG, Plantinga LC, et al. Association of residual urine output with mortality, quality of life, and inflammation in incident hemodialysis patients: the choices for healthy outcomes in caring for end-stage renal disease (CHOICE) study. Am J Kidney Dis. 2010; 56(2):348-358. doi:10.1053/j.ajkd.2010.03.020

[59] Suda T, Hiroshige K, Ohta T, et al. The contribution of residual renal function to overall nutritional status in chronic haemodialysis patients. Nephrol Dial Transplant. 2000; 15(3):396-401. doi:10.1093/ndt/15.3.396

[60] Vilar E, Wellsted D, Chandna SM, Greenwood RN, Farrington K. Residual renal function improves outcome in incremental haemodialysis despite reduced dialysis dose. Nephrol Dial Transplant. 2009; 24(8):2502-2510. doi:10.1093/ndt/gfp071

[61] Penne EL, van der Weerd NC, Grooteman MP, et al. Role of residual renal function in phosphate control and anemia management in chronic hemodialysis patients. Clin J Am Soc Nephrol. 2011; 6(2):281-289. doi:10.2215/CJN.04480510

[62] Wang AY, Wang M, Woo J, et al. Inflammation, residual kidney function, and cardiac hypertrophy are interrelated and combine adversely to enhance mortality and cardiovascular death risk of peritoneal dialysis patients. J. Am. Soc. Nephrol. 2004; 15(8):2186-2194. doi:10.1097/01.ASN.0000135053.98172.D6

[63] Palomo-Piñón S, Mora-Villalpando CJ, Del Carmen Prado-Uribe M, et al. Inflammation and myocardial damage markers influence loss of residual renal function in peritoneal dialysis patients. Arch Med Res. 2014; 45(6):484-488. doi:10.1016/j.arcmed.2014.07.003

[64] Selby NM, McIntyre CW. Peritoneal dialysis is not associated with myocardial stunning. Perit Dial Int. 2011; 31(1):27-33. PMID:20522673

[65] Panday VB, Tong ZP, Ng PL, et al. Dialysis modality and 2-year outcomes in patients with ischemic cardiomyopathy and end-stage renal disease. Int J Cardiol. 2014; 176(3):1097-1099. doi:10.1016/j.ijcard.2014.07.120

[66] Wang IK, Kung PT, Kuo WY, et al. Impact of dialysis modality on the survival of end-stage renal disease patients with or without cardiovascular disease. J Nephrol. 2013; 26(2):331-341. doi:10.5301/jn.5000149

[67] Locatelli F, Marcelli D, Conte F, et al. Survival and development of cardiovascular disease by modality of treatment in patients with end-stage renal disease. J Am Soc Nephrol. 2001; 12(11):2411-2417. doi:10.1681/ASN.V12112411

[68] Wang IK, Lu CY, Lin CL, et al. Comparison of the risk of de novo cardiovascular disease between hemodialysis and peritoneal dialysis patients with end-stage renal disease. Int J Cardiol. 2016; 218:219-224. doi:10.1016/j.ijcard.2016.05.036

[69] Vashistha T, Kalantar-Zadeh K, Molnar MZ, Torlén K, Mehrotra R. Dialysis modality and correction of uremic metabolic acidosis: relationship with all-cause and cause-specific mortality. Clin J Am Soc Nephrol. 2013; 8(2):254-264. doi:10.2215/CJN.05780612

[70] Raikou VD, Kyriaki D. Association between low serum bicarbonate concentrations and cardiovascular disease in patients in the end-stage of renal disease. Diseases. 2016; 4(4):36. doi:10.3390/diseases4040036

[71] Stenvinkel P. C-reactive protein: does it promote vascular disease? Nephrol Dial Transplant. 2006; 21(10):2718-2720. doi:10.1093/ndt/gfl317

[72] Amann K, Ritz C, Adamczak M, Ritz E. Why is coronary heart disease of uraemic patients so frequent and so devastating? Nephrol Dial Transplant. 2003; 18(4):631-640. doi:10.1093/ndt/gfg059

[73] Goodman W, Goldin J, Kuizon BD, et al. Coronary-artery calcification in young adults with end-stage renal disease who are undergoing dialysis. N Engl J Med. 2000; 342(20):1478-1483. doi:10.1056/NEJM200005183422003

[74] Barreto DV, Barreto FC, Carvalho AB, et al. Coronary calcification in hemodialysispatients: the contribution of traditional and uremia-related risk factors. Kidney Int. 2005; 67(4):1576-1582. doi:10.1111/j.1523-1755.2005.00239.x

[75] Charytan D, Kuntz RE, Mauri L, DeFilippi C. Distribution of coronary artery disease and relation to mortality in asymptomatic hemodialysis patients. Am J Kidney Dis. 2007; 49(3):409-416. doi:10.1053/j.ajkd.2006.11.042

[76] McCullough PA, Sandberg KP, Yee J, Hudson MP. Mortality benefit of angionensin-converting enzyme inhibitors after cardiac events in patients with end-stage renal disease. J Renin Angiotensin Aldosterone Syst. 2002; 3(3):188-191. doi:10.3317/jraas.2002.040

[77] Cice G, Ferrara L, Di Benedetto A, et al. Dilated cardiomyopathy in dialysis patients--beneficial effects of carvedilol: a double-blind, placebo-controlled trial. J Am Coll Cardiol. 2001; 37(2):407-411. doi:10.1016/s0735-1097(00)01158-x.

[78] Cice G, Ferrara L, D'Andrea A, et al. Carvedilol increases two-year survivalin dialysis patients with dilated cardiomyopathy: a prospective, placebo-controlled trial. J Am Coll Cardiol. 2003; 41(9):1438-1444. doi:10.1016/s0735-1097(03)00241-9.

[79] Baber U, Toto RD, de Lemos JA. Statins and cardiovascular risk reduction in patients with chronic kidney disease and end-stage renal disease. Am Heart Dis. 2007; 153(4):471-477. doi:10.1016/j.ahj.2006.10.042

[80] Wanner C, Tonelli M; Kidney Disease: improving global outcomes lipid guideline development work group members. KDIGO clinical practice guideline for lipid management in CKD: summary of recommendation statements and clinical approach to the patient. Kidney Int. 2014; 85(6):1303-1309. doi:10.1038/ki.2014.31.

[81] Yamamoto S, Yancey PG, Ikizler TA, et al. Dysfunctional high-density lipoprotein in patients on chronic hemodialysis. J Am Coll Cardiol. 2012; 60(23):2372-2379. doi:10.1016/j.jacc.2012.09.013.

[82] Zewinger S, Kleber ME, Rohrer L, et al. Symmetric dimethylarginine, high-density lipoproteins and cardiovascular disease. Eur Heart J. 2017; 38(20):1597-1607. doi:10.1093/eurheartj/ehx118.

[83] Liu JY, Birkmeyer NJ, Sanders JH, et al. Risks of morbidity and mortality in dialysis patients undergoing coronary artery bypass surgery. Circulation. 2000; 102(24):2973-2977. doi:10.1161/01.cir.102.24.2973

[84] US Renal Data System USRDS 2009 Annual Data Report: atlas of chronic kidney disease and end-stage renal disease in the United States, National Institutes of health, National Institute of diabetes and digestive and kidney diseases. Bethesda, MD, 2009.

[85] Green D, Roberts PR, New DI, Kalra PA. Sudden cardiac death in hemodialysis patients: an in-depth review. Am J Kidney Dis. 2011; 57(6):921-929. doi:10.1053/j.ajkd.2011.02.376.

[86] Bleyer AJ, Russell GB, Satko SG. Sudden and cardiac death rates in hemodialysis patients. Kidney Int. 1999; 55(4):1553-1559. doi:10.1046/j.1523-1755.1999.00391.x.

[87] Perl J., Chan C.T. Timing of sudden death relative to the hemodialysis procedure. Nat Clin Pract Nephrol. 2006; 2(12):668-669. doi:10.1038/ncpneph0345.

[88] Bauer A, Watanabe MA, Barthel P, et al. QRS duration and late mortality in unselected postinfarction patients of the revasculation era. Eur Heart J. 2006; 27(4):427-433. doi:10.1093/eurheartj/ehi683

[89] Block GA, Klassen PS, Lazarus JM, et al. Mineral metabolism, mortality and morbidity in maintenance hemodialysis. J Am Soc Nephrol. 2004; 15(8):2208-2218. doi:10.1097/01.ASN.0000133041.27682.A2

[90] Faul C, Amaral AP, Oskouei B, et al. FGF23 induces left ventricular hypertrophy. J Clin Invest. 2011; 121(11):4393-4408. doi:10.1172/JCI46122.

[91] Xie J, Yoon J, An SW, Kuro-o M, Huang CL. Soluble Klotho protects against uremic cardiomyopathy independently of fibroblast growth factor 23 and phosphate. J Am Soc Nephrol. 2015; 26(5):1150-1160. doi:10.1681/ASN.2014040325.

[92] Hyperphosphataemia in chronic kidney disease. Management of hyperphosphataemia in patients with stage 4 or 5 chronic kidney disease. National Institute for Health and Clinical Excellence (UK). NICE clinical guideline No 157; March 2013.

[93] Shanahan CM, Crouthamel MH, Kapustin A, Giachelli CM. Arterial calcification in chronic kidney disease: key roles for calcium and phosphate. Circ Res. 2011; 109(6):697-711. doi:10.1161/CIRCRESAHA.110.234914.

[94] Mizobuchi M, Towler D, Slatopolsky E. Vascular calcification: the killer of patients with chronic kidney disease. J Am Soc Nephrol. 2009; 20(7):1453-1464. doi:10.1681/ASN.2008070692.

[95] Guérin AP, London GM, Marchais SJ, Metivier F. Arterial stiffening and vascular calcifications in end-stage renal disease. Nephrol Dial Transplant. 2000; 15(7):1014-1021. doi:10.1093/ndt/15.7.1014.

[96] Toussaint ND, Kerr PG. Vascular calcification and arterial stiffness in chronic kidney disease: implications and management. Nephrology (Carlton). 2007; 12(5):500-509. doi:10.1111/j.1440-1797.2007.00823.x.

[97] Van den Bergh G, Opdebeeck B, D'Haese PC, Verhulst A. The vicious cycle of arterial stiffness and arterial media calcification. Trends Mol Med. 2019; 25(12):1133-1146. doi:10.1016/j.molmed.2019.08.006.

[98] Rong S, Qiu X, Jin X, et al. Risk factors for heart valve calcification in chronic kidney disease. Medicine (Baltimore). 2018; 97(5):e9804. doi:10.1097/MD.0000000000009804

[99] Raggi P. Cardiovascular disease: Coronary artery calcification predicts risk of CVD in patients with CKD. Nat Rev Nephrol. 2017; 13(6):324-326. doi:10.1038/nrneph.2017.61.

[100] Gauthier-Bastien A, Ung RV, Larivière R, et al. Vascular remodeling and media calcification increases arterial stiffness in chronic kidney disease. Clin Exp Hypertens. 2014; 36(3):173-180. doi:10.3109/10641963.2013.804541.

[101] Sprague SM. A comparative review of the efficacy and safety of established

phosphate binder: calcium, sevelamer, and lanthanum carbonate. Curr Med Res Opin. 2007; 23(12):3167-3175. doi:10.1185/030079907X242719

[102] Patel L, Bernard LM, Elder GJ. Sevelamer versus calcium-based binders for treatment of hyperphosphatemia in CKD: a meta-analysis of randomized controlled trials. Clin J Am Soc Nephrol. 2016; 11(2):232-244. doi:10.2215/CJN.06800615

[103] Floege J, Covic AC, Ketteler M, et al. A phase III study of the efficacy and safety of a novel iron-based phosphate binder in dialysis patients. Kidney Int. 2014; 86(3):638-647. doi:10.1038/ki.2014.58

[104] Komaba H, Taniguchi M, Wada A, et al. Parathyroidectomy and survival among Japanese hemodialysis patients with secondary hyperparathyroidism. Kidney Int. 2015; 88(2):350-359. doi:10.1038/ki.2015.72

[105] Chertow GM, Block GA, Correa-Rotter R, et al; EVOLVE Trial Investigators. Effect of cinacalcet on cardiovascular disease in patients undergoing dialysis. New Engl J Med. 2012; 387(26):2482-2494. doi:10.1056/NEJMoa1205624

[106] Wheeler DC, London GM, Parfrey PS, et al; EValuationOf Cinacalcet HCl Therapy to Lower Cardio Vascular Events (EVOLVE) Trial Investigators. Effects of cinacalcet on atherosclerotic and nonatherosclerotic cardiovascular events in patients receiving hemodialysis: the evaluation of cinacalcet HCL therapy to lower cardiovascular events (EVOLVE) trial. J Am Heart Assoc. 2014; 3(6):e001363. doi:10.1161/JAHA.114.001363

[107] Chung DR, Huh K. Novel pandemic influenza A (H1N1) and community associated methicillin resistant Staphylococcus aureus pneumonia. Expert Rev Anti Infect Ther. 2015; 13(2):197-207. doi:10.1586/14787210.2015.999668

[108] Moreillon P, Que YA. Infective endocarditis. Lancet. 2004; 363(9403):139-149. doi:10.1016/S0140-6736(03)15266-X

[109] Fowler VG, Miro JM, Hoen B, et al. Staphylococcus aureus endocarditis: a consequence of medical progress. JAMA. 2005; 293(24):3012-3021. doi:10.1001/jama.293.24.3012

[110] Ezekowyz JA, McAlister FA, Armstrong PW. Anemia is common in heart failure and is associated with pooroutcomes: insights from a cohort of 12 065 patients with new-onset heart failure. Circulation. 2003; 107(2): 223-225. doi:10.1161/01.cir.0000052622.51963.fc

[111] Philipp S, Ollmann H, Schimk T, et al. The impact of anemia and kidney function in congestive heart failure and preserved systolic function. Nephrol Dial Transplant. 2005; 20(5):915-919. doi:10.1093/ndt/gfh753

[112] Fishbane S. Erythropoiesis-stimulating agent treatment with full anemia correction: a new perspective. Kidney Int. 2009; 75(4):358-365. doi:10.1038/ki.2008.467

[113] Haase VH. Hypoxia-inducible factor-prolyl hydroxylase inhibitors in the treatment of anemia of chronic kidney disease. Kidney Int Suppl (2011). 2021; 11(1):8-25. doi:10.1016/j.kisu.2020.12.002

[114] Nakhoul F, Yigla M, Gilman R, Reisner SA, Abassi Z. The pathogenesis of pulmonary hypertension in haemodialysis patients via arterio-venous access. Nephrol Dial Transplant. 2005; 20(8):1686-1692. doi:10.1093/ndt/gfh840

[115] Von Bibra H, Castro L, Autenrieth G, McLeod A, Gurland HJ.

The effects of arteriovenous shunts on cardiac function in renal dialysis patients – an echocardiographic evaluation. Clin Nephrol. 1978; 9(5):205-209. PMID:657597

[116] Yigla M, Nakhoul F, Sabag A, et al. Pulmonary hypertension in patients with end-stage renal disease. Chest. 2003; 123(5):1577-1582. doi:10.1378/chest.123.5.1577

[117] Clarkson MR, Giblin L, Brown A, Little D, Donohoe J. Reversal of pulmonary hypertension after ligation of a brachiocephalic arteriovenous fistula. Am J Kidney Dis. 2002; 40(3):E8. doi:10.1053/ajkd.2002.34932

[118] Yigla M, Abassi Z, Reisner SA, Nakhoul F. Pulmonary hypertension in hemodialysis patients: an unrecognized threat. Semin Dial. 2006; 19(5):353-357. doi:10.1111/j.1525-139X.2006.00186.x

[119] Crowley SD, Butterly DW, Peter RH, Schwab SJ. Coronary steal from a left internal mammary artery coronary artery bypass graft by a left upper extremity ateriovenous hemodialysis fistula. Am J Kidney Dis. 2002; 40(4):852-855. doi:10.1053/ajkd.2002.35701